Our Dementia Diary
Irene, Alzheimer's and Me

Rachael Dixey

Our Dementia Diary
Irene, Alzheimer's and Me

Published by
Medina Publishing Ltd.
310 Ewell Road
Surbiton
Surrey KT6 7AL
medinapublishing.com

ISBN Hardback: 978-1-909339-73-6
ISBN Kindle: 978-1-909339-74-3

Printed and bound by Interak Printing House, Poland

CIP Data: A catalogue record of this book is available from the British Library

Our Dementia Diary
Irene, Alzheimer's and Me

Rachael Dixey

Medina Publishing

Contents

Prologue

Irene, Alzheimer's and me – Alzheimer's came between us. It does that,
drives you and the love of your life apart, going your separate ways because
you cannot follow. That's the story really, that's it. The end.

Or that's the condensed version. The long version is what follows.
This is a true story.

Part One: Beginnings

Irene

Irene was an actress, a comedienne, not by profession but by instinct. When I first met her she was a vital member of the village amateur dramatics society. She played the Mother in *Barefoot in the Park*, Helena in *A Midsummer Night's Dream* and, when she came on as the Runcible Spoon in *The Owl and the Pussycat*, a child in the audience piped up in a loud voice, 'She's a tall lady!' Indeed she was, made taller and thinner in a sheaf of metallic blue with a large spoon shape like a cowl hovering over her head. She could deliver Joyce Grenfell's line 'George, don't do that!' to great comic effect. I'm biased, but she really was wonderful on stage. Other times, usually when we'd had friends round for dinner and were slumped on sofas, she would go out to make coffee then pop her head round the living room door and use her own unseen arm to wrap it round her neck, in the pretence that someone was trying to kidnap her. I always knew what was coming, had seen it dozens of times, but it was always funny. So the sense of fun hung around Irene like a charm. She larked about, it was in her nature.

By profession she was an English teacher. It's what she had always wanted to be from childhood, having adored her English teacher at secondary school. They developed such a close relationship that the teacher left Irene all her books when she died. I imagine Irene herself was an inspirational teacher, especially good with troubled lads and enthusing generations of girls. Irene loved literature, she inspired people to read, she could quote poetry, she loved to discuss the latest good read, or what was on the Booker list. She loved

Wordsworth and she took me to see Shakespeare plays in Stratford. She put on a production of *Macbeth* when she was teaching in Singapore (what her young Chinese and Malay charges made of the three witches or of Scottish internecine plotting, who knows). She would ride around the humid streets of Singapore on her bicycle, long hair streaming behind.

Although she was an exhibitionist, she had no pretensions and told stories at her own expense. Like the story of her first and only meeting with her heroine, the great Doris Lessing, in London. Irene stayed a night with a former pupil, now grown up and lodging with Lessing, who liked to house budding young writers. Doris came in and was introduced to Irene, said, 'Oh, hello,' showed no further interest in her whatsoever, merely turning to Irene's friend and asking, 'Have you seen the cat?' She had the two largest, sleekest, best-fed cats Irene had ever seen. How she laughed at the idea that she might have held any interest for Lessing, though she secretly hoped for some sort of insightful discussion about literature.

Irene also told the story of joining a choir and how the dissatisfied leader had asked them to repeat the same verse over and over, eventually demanding, 'Can we try that again please, but without Irene?'

Singapore, for VSO, was her first real sojourn abroad. Later, she had another big adventure, as the brains behind raising the money to buy two Land Rovers for Save the Children Fund. She and three chums drove the Land Rovers to Burkina Faso in the mid-1970s, across the Sahara in the days when there was no tarred road. The foursome had split there, Irene travelling down through Ghana and on to Ethiopia, where she taught in a secondary school. One of the many revolutions, with its associated indiscriminate killings, divided the expatriate community into those who wanted to stay and those who wanted to leave. Stepping over bodies in the street on the way to work finally tipped the balance for Irene and she returned to England, finding work fairly easily in the late 1970s and in time to meet me in 1980.

She was a close friend of a friend of mine and for a short while we would go out as a threesome. Only when the mutual friend was ill one night and Irene and I went together to a film did I realise we were attracted to each other. After the film – *Being There* with Peter Sellers and Shirley MacLaine – we went to a party. I can still remember sitting in a chair with Irene cross-legged on the floor by my feet, gazing up at me with what I realised with a jolt was an expression of love. It was strange, as our first impressions had been quite different – I thought she was a spoilt prankster and she thought I was stuffy and stuck up. How wrong can you be?

We got together and thereafter celebrated 22 October as our anniversary. My memory of that first autumn of being madly in love is of golden leaves and blue skies – those marvellous crisp, not-too-cold days we get in October. That song with the line 'But I miss you most of all, my darling, when autumn leaves start to fall' hits me hard.

We knew pretty quickly that we would spend our lives together, though I can remember standing in her little terraced house and each agreeing to make do with the other until someone else came along. She really wanted children and I had plans to return overseas. I was 26, she 33. In the event, we bought a house, opened a joint bank account, shared all our money and somehow jumped into what felt like our destiny. Later, we would open each other's mail and finish each other's sentences. Some people baulk at the phrase 'my other half' – I do myself – but when you do find a great love, it really feels like that, that you are only half of something. We were a very 'coupley' couple because it just felt right. We also rebelled against it at times, that knowledge that our lives were destined to be intertwined, because it takes away the possibility of any other way of life. But really we just settled into it; comfortable, companionable and loving each other deeply. We enjoyed the same things, so we did them together. People used to get our names mixed up – some still do, and apologise, as if it upsets me. It doesn't. It's kind of nice.

We did have rows, blazing ones – I once threw a mug at Irene, my favourite one too, and it smashed – but I now have no idea what they were about. I do know that Irene was always the first to come round, always the one to seek reconciliation. We also both knew that the final recourse for any couple, the threat to leave, was never open to us for we both knew neither of us ever would.

We came from the same social background, born into the post-War generation. Our mothers were both habitual margarine tub hoarders and make-doers, enterprising women with intelligence that wasn't properly harnessed in the stay-at-home 1950s. Our fathers left school early but studied at night school to get qualifications. My father read Dickens in the evenings; hers could recite long passages of poetry. We were what used to be called respectable working class, where our parents were intimidated by the confident middle classes, didn't mix with people who were 'common' (those who chewed gum and said ain't), and knew education was important even if they couldn't really help us with our homework. Later, having got to university, we both morphed into people who had lunch and dinner instead of dinner and tea. All four parents were liberal people with social consciences. I don't know what they went through privately when we came out, but to us they were only ever accepting. My mother loved Irene and Irene stood up to her in ways that I never dared. There were many happy times with both sets of parents.

Irene was an extrovert. Five feet-ten with long, lithe legs and blue-grey eyes, at 40 she dyed her hair a shade of blonde, saying she wanted more fun and blondes seemed to have it. When still only in her early forties, she had to give up school teaching. It was a huge blow, but her hearing loss and tinnitus made school a nightmare environment. She wasn't suited to life outside an institution, was not a self-starter, so after doing an MA in Victorian literature, followed by a half-hearted attempt at writing a novel, she started to teach English Literature classes for adults. She loved the interaction, the discussion, the stimulation. I suspect she also loved being the centre of attraction of a group of women (her students were mainly women) who thought she was marvellous. But Irene was more complicated and I saw a side to her that others did not see. She could get depressed, wondering what life was all about. She had high moral principles and would criticize herself for wanting to run for God. And by that she didn't mean enter some marathon or other, rather that she took the troubles of the world on her shoulders as if she could sort them all out. At times I would have to coax her to be sociable, but once we were out at some gathering she would be the life and soul. She could be loud.

We did the usual things that a university-educated, reasonably well-off, left wing-ish, feminist couple did: saw friends and family, pursued our careers; went on holiday to Scotland or France, trekked in the high Alps; saw the latest films, read the latest books; cooked, walked, camped, canoed. We laughed a lot. Our lives went by quite happily with no major dramas. For Irene, the adjustment to not working full time in a school was the biggest thing we'd had to deal with – and it was big. We had a six-month stint in the United States during that time and did some incredible wilderness walking; our lives really centred on our holidays, always poring over maps and plotting where we'd go next. We planned for me to retire at 55 so that we could do more of just having fun. We learned to sail too, with the thought that one day we would just sail away.

Alzheimer's teaches you to take nothing for granted. Although we planned to grow old together we never took our relationship for granted – we somehow always worked at it, which is maybe why it lasted. She was the best judge of character I've ever met, and generous with her affection. That she loved me I never doubted, with a deep, unconditional love that never wavered. She used to say, 'Come here, you gorgeous fascinating creature.' She said it often and although I said it less, my love for her was returned in equal measure.

I wrote in my journal in 2008:

> When I first met Irene, we knew we would spend our lives together and we have, very happily. We grew to be like two old trees, strong individuals on the surface, but with our roots totally intertwined underneath, me inconceivable without her. Sometimes in moments of coherence, Irene will still say, 'I am you and you are me,' which says it all.
>
> Even after more than 20-plus years, my heart and eyes would light up whenever I saw her. They still do, but there are all sorts of more complex feelings there too now. To know that we matter profoundly to another person is the core and purpose of our lives, and dementia robs us of the certainty of knowing whether I still matter profoundly to Irene – does she kiss everyone's hand too, or is it reserved for me? I believe she still does know who I am, and that anyone with dementia has an emotional memory which remains after other types of memory have gone. And her eyes light up still, for the moment.

So, that's the picture of Irene and me. I'm not far off 60 now so we've had each other at the centre of our lives for most of our adult years. No wonder I'm the last person that Irene recognizes, which is a privilege and a comfort.

Why Write About Us?

Why write this book? Why do I want to pour my heart out in public, wash the dirty linen, produce one of those ouch-making misery memoires that somehow reduces the author? I could call it Fifty Shades of Dementia but it would be more like fifty shades of black. A depressing read for everyone? Not depressing, but certainly sad, while it marvels at the wonder of love that two people can feel for each other, that such love is possible. So it's a happy story but…it's about a person who ceases to be what she might have been, and confirms the truism that loss is the price of love.

A book like this has to be more than a cathartic outpouring of grief and loss, an attempt to heal a deep wound that the popular media tells us might lead to 'closure' but that the counsellors suggest could at least lead to living a more normal life. It might help to leave behind the huge emotional baggage that's like a millstone around your neck as you drown. Maybe writing turns that millstone into a lodestone, somehow swinging you around, reorienting you, launching you in a new direction – or at least leaving you feeling anchored, magnetically attached and grounded. What motivates me, apart from the sense that I can do it, is that so many books have helped me – cheesy perhaps, but true. Would I have wanted to read someone else's outpourings about Alzheimer's? Someone who had really been there, lived it, lost the love of their life to this disease? Yes, I would have wanted that book, would have sought it out. Something to rescue me as I helplessly watched the woman I loved, my partner, my soul mate, diminishing and being diminished.

I gorged myself on books when I had cancer. Lance Armstrong, *It's Not About the Bike* and *C: Because Cowards Get Cancer Too*, John Diamond's book about his battle with throat cancer. Armstrong survived (OK, he was a cheat), Diamond didn't. I'm alive, I'm well. Buttressed by books, I will survive losing the love of my life to early onset dementia.

Although our losses are so different, I still devoured Joan Didion's memoir *The Year of Magical Thinking*, written after her husband dropped dead from a heart attack. Her loss was sudden, dramatic, definitive, all or nothing. Mine was slow-motion, ambiguous, indecisive. A slow descent into fog, not a sudden blackout. Joan Didion describes the event then talks of other things, then lopes back to the dreadful moment, over and over, as if doing so will somehow make her believe it. A year of magical thinking – magical perhaps meaning dreamlike rather than enchanted; a blur, a dream, but one you don't wake up from, no matter how much you try to shake yourself.

Someone remarked that John Bayley's trilogy about his wife Iris Murdoch was disappointing, that there wasn't enough about the great Iris. Even so, it's perhaps the best known writing about the experience of living with a partner who has Alzheimer's. For Iris, one of the most brilliant minds, it was a spectacular fall. Alzheimer's is nothing if not a great leveller. But most people are not like the great Iris Murdoch. Bayley's books are inevitably as much, if not more, about him than about her. I'm not a novelist, I'm not even a writer. If this book seems to be centred on me it's because I can't help it. This is my reality. If it helps just one person get through the nightmare it will have been worth it.

November 2012   I am in Deia, Mallorca. I have come here to get away and also to face it all. It was recommended by someone I trust, who thought it would suit me, the place to string together a book or at least be creative. It's also, I discover, the place where Robert Graves lived and where he wrote, the guidebook says, some of his 'finest love poems'. It seems a suitable place then, to be writing about a theme that is so common – finding a great love, and losing it. It is the basic story (Irene used to say there were only ever seven themes and every story ever written is a variation on one of them). Graves also had dementia, we learn from a devastating sentence in a biographer's footnote:

In the 1970s his productivity fell off; and the last decade of his life was lost in silence and senility.

I did have a vague recollection that Robert Graves is famous for *I, Claudius* but more so for *Goodbye to All That* and that seems more appropriate than ever – because even after only being here for one day I understand that it is what I want to do   to say goodbye to all that, to Alzheimer's and loss.

I have this burden of the unsaid. In that respect, I have something in common with Joan Didion in that a sudden death also robs you of the opportunity to say goodbye. Dementia means that the things you should say to the one you are losing will be forever unsaid. Irene left without saying goodbye to anything – our life, our home. She was here, and then she was gone. I have never said goodbye, never talked to her about the fact that we have to be apart, never talked to her about her illness, never done the things you would if someone had cancer – like in *Calendar Girls*, the poignant scene on the moor, sitting side by side in the Land Rover, looking out and saying what needed to be said to each other. 'Look – I'm not going to make it – you will have to carry on but I will always love you.' And, 'I know . . . I don't want you to go but I will always love you too and we had the most wonderful life together. Thank you for all the great times and for being my soul mate, my loyal soul mate and my love.' We have so much of our life still here, in our house, all our things, souvenirs, photos, and only me wandering around in it, listening to the radio so there's another presence in the house, trying to make a life here for one. What would I have said? The book helps to say those things.

Of course, there was a lot of talk between us about her problems, and there's a danger that it becomes all you talk about – how to manage, how to help, going over the anxieties of the day, coaxing, cajoling, trying to make the other feel better. If you're not careful, in the end the person can feel they really are a problem, and there are times when you just have to get on, try to have a good time, forget about it for a while, get used to a new normal. And when the one with dementia gets to a certain stage of unawareness of their condition, it gets easier, what I've called, irreverently, the happy clappy stage.

Memory is not a huge set of computer files that we can call up at will; lots of things I can't remember at all. There are events I can't recall going to, let alone what happened there. And our memory is partial anyway: I cannot remember conversations but I can remember how to get somewhere, even if I've only been there once. My memory is spatial, Irene's was verbal. She could remember whole conversations from years ago and, ironically, her memory was better than mine. Another thing lost along with Irene, the recollections. I had no one to share my joint memories with, our shared life was mine alone, and I could no longer ask her about events dimly remembered. So in terms of what I wrote in the immediacy of the moment – I cannot tinker with that in either its form or content. It will have to do.

I would come home perhaps from seeing Irene, and have to write. Or I would feel a great tide of grief, and writing somehow kept it from washing me away. These jottings form a sort of diary, of that moment, that day, and are presented in the book chronologically, with a few interpolations to make sense of it all. I also wrote summaries of what was happening, such as my dealings with social services. Much of it was so unbelievable that unless I had recorded it people would think my memory faulty. I was asked to write a couple of small pieces for the Alzheimer's Society LGBT (Lesbian, Gay, Bisexual and Transgendered) newsletter. Thus I have a motley collection from which to piece together the story. Well, not the whole story, as the story hasn't ended yet. But, a bit like knowing the ending of Titanic, the reader will know there will be a gradual sinking, that for Irene at least there will be no happy ending, so it doesn't really matter if I give it away.

My ramblings will make sense to anyone else on a dementia journey, little sparks of recognition, shared tragedies or moments when you just have to laugh. I connect with stories on the radio, in the paper, on television, about early onset dementia but have never read a book about it. And it makes no difference that we are a same-sex couple: our story is the same as any other couple's wherein love resides. Those lucky enough to have found a soul mate must inevitably suffer a loss

Alzheimer's

This book isn't just about the oldest story – finding love and losing it. It's also a lot about Alzheimer's and what it's like to have it, to care for someone with it, and to lose the love of your life to it. Would it earn the title of the cruellest disease? Maybe, but that's not the point; all losses and undignified diseases are cruel and all pernicious, taking us to the point beyond which words are adequate.

Alzheimer's. It's only now, writing this in Deia in 2012 that I realise I haven't a clue what Alzheimer's is, or who Alzheimer was. I have no real idea about what it does to a person's brain – haven't wanted to know, as how can you bear the details of your loved one's brain being turned to mush, of knowing precisely which cells, proteins, synapses or whatever neurological is happening? I have heard that after a post mortem, the brain of an Alzheimer's patient looks like a cauliflower. And it's not meant to look like that. I don't even have the terminology of the brain, always forget about stuff like the hippocampus and only know that the frontal lobes must be somewhere near the front. Do I want to know?

Frau Auguste Deter was the first person to be diagnosed with the disease that was to be named after Dr Alzheimer. It was 1901; she died five years later in 1906. She was 51 when she was diagnosed, about the same age as Irene was when we first began to worry about the symptoms; at 57 Irene had received the diagnosis beyond doubt. I can imagine Irene's brain scan with large decayed blobs highlighted in red, like one of those infra-red pictures which show where your body is losing heat. In the years from 1906, when Alzheimer's was first recognized and labelled, to 2004, when Irene was diagnosed, there doesn't seem to be any advance on preventing it, stopping it – it seems all we can do is see it better.

Irene could have had a disease called after any number of clinicians working in the heady days of discovery at the turn of the 19th century. It was the psychiatrist Kraeplin who first described a distinctive type of dementia with organic changes caused by a disease agent. He could have called it after any one of a number of colleagues – Fischer, Fuller, Perusini – but instead chose Dr Alzheimer.

Kraeplin was the ambitious head of an academic department based in Munich and in the tenth edition of his definitive work in 1910, *Psychiatrie*, he included Alzheimer's study of Frau Auguste D. After her death, her brain was sent to Alzheimer, who identified the plaques and fibrils that had led to her disorientation, paranoia, unpredictable behaviour and profound cognitive impairment. The autopsy showed that around a third of cortical cells had died. It was considered a new disease because although it looked like the senile dementia found in older people's brains, this disease could start as early as the age of 40 and there was clearly a disease process occurring – the causes of which are still being unravelled.

There have recently been suggestions about junk food and its links with the rise in Alzheimer's. Irene had a great diet, ate healthily, and in 1996, much to my amazement, gave up eating meat. When John Gummer fed his daughter a beefburger, Irene declared, 'They can bloody well lie to everyone else, but they are not lying to me!' With that, and the media frenzy about mad cow disease, she turned her back on beef sandwiches, bacon, pork chops, steaks. This is someone who managed to get through her steak tartare in France somewhere, just to see what it was and not realising it was raw; someone for whom one of my greatest acts of devotion (as a confirmed vegetarian since 1969) was to go to our local butcher to buy her favourite cuts. I was stunned by her conversion, and she kept to it too, until later, in her care home, it seemed that the best thing was to give her as many calories as possible, keep things simple, and so she started to munch whatever was on the menu, and she didn't know anyway what she was eating. So, a link between Alzheimer's and junk food? Maybe not in Irene's case.

George Monbiot has an article in the *Guardian* exploring the links between Type 2 diabetes and Alzheimer's. It seems that insulin-like growth factors are much lower in the brains of those with Alzheimer's. Insulin in the brain functions to promote plasticity, growth and survival of nerve cells; it helps to regulate signals from one nerve cell to another. And of course, the next day there is a flood of letters to say that George Monbiot has got it sort of right...but things are much more complicated than that.

I pause, defeated by the complexity of my brain's chemistry, marvelling at how it can write this while listening to the radio, simultaneously taking in the weather, looking out at the countryside, and all this is going on in my brain, tapping out the letters on my keyboard, letters learnt in childhood. Well, this is a memoir, not a scientific treatise – the misery is top quality, the facts and figures might be dodgy. But I do know all about the effect on behaviour, the effect on personality, the slow destruction of both. I do know that the scan led the psychiatrist to conclude that the only explanation for Irene's problems was Alzheimer's, so it was visible, measurable – obvious.

Alzheimer himself died in 1915 of that most prosaic illness, tonsillitis, at the age of 51.

The Beginnings

Lots of people ask me what the first signs of Irene's dementia were. I suspect they are asking because a little worm of worry is gnawing away at them about themselves, or someone they know. I can only say it's not about having to write lists in case you would forget things. (If you have the sense to write lists, you're probably OK.) This often produces relief in the questioner and they murmur appreciatively and move the conversation along. Sometimes they really do want to know, and it's only with hindsight that I can give some kind of answer. I think Alzheimer's was making its presence felt as early as 1999 but we didn't know it. Irene then was 52.

The first sign is perhaps a strange detachment, as if that person has shrink-wrapped their responses to what's around them. There's a faltering in sharpness, and discussions lose their sparkle and wit. There's anxiety and a reduction in confidence. People misplace things a little too often. It's perhaps one of the most unsettling stages, like when the speech and lip movements are only slightly out of synch in a film. It doesn't really matter, but it's irritating.

Is this what they mean by early signs? If you then rushed in to do crosswords and played Scrabble every day, would it halt the relentless march of brain damage? They seem to have found evidence that doing word puzzles every day wards off dementia. Irene used to do the cryptic *Guardian* crossword – admittedly she didn't always finish it, but we regularly sent in the slightly easier *Observer* crossword, though we never won a prize. It was when I started to get the clues before she did that I realized something was indeed wrong. But I don't think doing those crosswords helped one little bit in staving it off.

The beginning, then, is blurry because for so long the symptoms didn't seem that different from what many fiftysomethings are going through, the jokes about going upstairs and forgetting what you've gone for. But dementia isn't just about memory, it's about your ability to think, about all cognition. So Irene not only forgot where things belonged in the kitchen, she'd also lose the sense of sequence, so she no longer knew how to follow a recipe. It became clearer that Irene's problems in coping with daily life were not just to do with being disorganised, being hard of hearing or losing confidence. Her driving skills were going – and this was someone who knew how to double declutch and could drive a Land Rover up a sandbank. She was working part time with adults, running literature classes, and she literally began to lose the plot – not only could she not remember a story, she couldn't understand it. One day she asked me to read the end of a book, as she couldn't make sense of it, and she was teaching a class on it the next day. She'd always been a teacher and had so much experience to fall back on, but this was deserting her. I suspect that her students, mainly older women, saw these changes and accommodated them with kindness – she was too popular for them not to.

We went to see the film *Iris*, a moving evocation of the decline of Iris Murdoch. We left the cinema in silence, sharing an unspoken understanding that it somehow related to us.

Looking back, I can see that Irene's reaction to my diagnosis of cancer in 2001 was strangely muted. That diagnosis came on a day that is seared into most people's brains – 11 September 2001, now known simply as 9/11. Irene sat in the waiting room as I was getting my results – results which confirmed what we'd suspected a week earlier, so it wasn't entirely news. The TV screen told Irene what was happening in New York, and it occupied me during that strange day. I sat mesmerized, as most people were, and could only be thankful that I was alive, even if I did have cancer. But Irene had asked if it was OK if she went out as she had envelopes to deliver in the village, for a cancer charity as it happened. At the time I thought it a bit odd that she didn't stay in with me, but we're both pragmatists and I'd said that I was fine and anyway she wasn't going to be long. Later, through my long treatment, she was there for me but somehow not always keyed in. At the time, you don't jump straight to thinking it could be dementia – nothing so dramatic, of course not. I put it all down to shock, her way of dealing with it, and she was a good, kind and patient nurse for that year. With hindsight, though, I can begin to interpret her behaviour and reactions, put them into context.

In November 2003, at my suggestion, she saw our GP, a kind man who arranged for Irene to see a psychologist. Initial tests suggested there was cause for concern. For a while Irene enjoyed seeing someone called Sue, but was angry when she felt Sue had dumped her, saying that all she'd wanted was data for her research. I can't confirm the truth of this: at that stage, Irene was independently driving herself to appointments. Each stage led to the need for further investigation rather than the hoped-for reassurance that really we were the 'worried well'. Irene needed a brain scan, which finally took place in January 2004. She caused havoc as she pulled the orange emergency cord in the loo – twice. Obviously she was discombobulated by the experience. The nurse on duty was most displeased – an extraordinary reaction in a situation where disturbed and distressed people were presumably routine. The nurse shouted at Irene, and I in turn gave her a piece of my mind.

After anxious months waiting for the scan results, in early April 2004 we finally got to see the consultant. He took me off to one room and asked me my perception of Irene's problems while Irene was given the usual battery of tests. Then we both sat down with him and he explained his verdict. Alzheimer's, he thought, was the only explanation. Irene was 56.

Even now, so many years on, I can put myself exactly back in that room and feel the reaction I had then. This was the nightmare coming true. It was like an electric shock. The consultant was not particularly skilled, it seemed to me, at handling such dreadful news. Irene and I both swung into denial mode and started to dispute his diagnosis. He seemed to have no rejoinder.. Soon, we were outside the revolving doors of this impressive new psychiatric hospital, disbelieving and bewildered. Somehow I drove home.

Even on the pavement outside the hospital, Irene firmly dismissed the verdict and decided she wanted to move on with her life, to put 'that horrible man' behind her. She'd found the testing demeaning and confidence-sapping. The tone was set: we never used the A word again, never again talked about it, except once, much later, when she was so far beyond comprehension that it didn't matter. By then the word held no horror for her.

I spoke about it to no one. A few days later we set off for a scheduled week in Mallorca and, in my memory, we had a good time. Irene felt a lot happier now that she had decided to put all the testing behind her, but my emotions were all over the place. Moreover, I knew I had started on a journey where, for the first time in our partnership, I was keeping things from Irene. In respecting her coping mechanism of denial, I was unable to share the burden with her. The consultant said we'd get a follow-up with one of his staff. This finally came in August, a good four months after the diagnosis.

After that first appointment Irene declined to see anyone and I decided to go along with this – I couldn't force her, after all. I was still uncertain that this was the true diagnosis, dredging up other possible causes in some kind of optimistic collusion with Irene. Even now, I still feel let down by the length of the process, notwithstanding Irene's reluctance to engage. Having to wait several months for the results of a brain scan isn't good enough! Neither is waiting another several months for a 'follow-up appointment'.

By early in 2005, while still trying to pretend there might be nothing really wrong, I recognised I needed help with it all. I saw my GP in February, motivated to go because, in the space of a week, four separate friends and family members had had a quiet word with me. Each had concluded that Irene really wasn't right, that her behaviour was beyond 'slightly worrying'. They were as worried about the strain on me as they were about Irene. I guess they sensed a mass cover-up. In place of murmured sympathy, the nice young woman GP we'd seen before was blunt. She predicted that in three or four years' time Irene would be in residential care. I was stunned. Stupidly, I tried to carry on in to work but instead ended up crying on the sofa of friends in our village.

I was actually grateful for the GP's honest confirmation. I'd carried the secret for too long. Yes, I'd talked to people about Irene's memory, sought their views, but the actual diagnosis I had kept to myself. And any secret corrodes from within, makes you both weary and wary, as the holding in and holding back becomes a default position. The energy it takes to do this means you can go off like a volcano when it all gets too much. Any gay person knows this, which is why being out is such a relief. So I set about telling people, firstly Irene's brother Gordon and then our families. I outed Irene as a person with Alzheimer's.

Later that year, when the GP hadn't offered to follow up, or to see Irene or to refer us to anyone (maybe they wait until people come forward, or maybe this is how they manage a large caseload), I sought an appointment with the original psychiatrist who had given us the verdict. I went along with Irene's closest friend, Barbara, the one who had introduced us. I can barely remember what we talked about, except that he confirmed his opinion. He also said that the life expectancy of someone with Alzheimer's is eight or nine years. Barbara and I reeled out to catch the bus home. The only seats free were at the front facing backwards, which meant we had an audience of all the other passengers. We were lachrymose and stunned. Barbara said softly, 'Let's not talk for a bit'.

As an assertive middle-class professional, I could refer myself to the appropriate clinical psychologist. She involved a community psychiatric nurse (CPN) from the 'younger people with dementia' team, who agreed to see Irene at home. The clinical psychologist was surprised at this self-referral, but it was obvious that we needed help so I was 'in'. It was a relief. Irene by then was in a state where it was easy to explain the presence of professionals by simply saying they were there to help. Irene no longer had the capacity to ask relevant questions, had lost insight. This started a long period of the CPN coming out around once a month and seeing us at home, a process that continued until Irene was admitted to hospital in August 2007. She balanced professionalism, personal concern, huge experience, insight and friendliness in a way that was perfect. She probably earns less than she needs to keep a family, an unsung hero. At times she brought with her a consultant psychiatrist, also a lovely woman, and Irene often made them both laugh. She would also sit there meekly while we discussed her case. I had evolved into a carer, a shift that was necessary but so painful in such a previously equal partnership.

Somewhere around this time we saw a solicitor and did the enduring power of attorney paperwork. I explained to Irene that it was something we ought to do, which she cheerfully accepted. We were familiar with solicitors because as a same-sex couple in the days before civil partnerships, we did not have the legal protection afforded to married couples. We did the paperwork so that I would have power of attorney for Irene, and she for me –a false symmetry but one which served the purpose.

Despite my relentless cheerfulness and my ability to summon up reserves to keep going, I realise, looking back, my mood was low for many years as we had run out of conversation. Irene could not initiate it or sustain it and her ability to converse had become so basic that I was bored. That sounds terrible and it is terrible.

So that's the bare story. That's how Alzheimer's arrived in our lives, as it does in so many people's lives.

Notes for Irene's Helpers

The years leading up to a dementia diagnosis are tough, full of uncertainty. You've that unsettling feeling that things aren't quite right but not majorly wrong either. Later, all hell breaks loose. We had just over three years of progressive worsening. The rest of 2004 was sort of OK. 2005, more difficult. 2006, the shit hit the fan. I hate that crude expression but it fits the bill.

Increasingly Irene could not be on her own. By September 2006, I needed a rota of paid helpers and friends in order that she would not be alone for more than half an hour at any time. This was more psychological – she needed company. The physical safety that everyone mentions didn't seem as important and, as our CPN said, lots of people with quite advanced dementia seem to manage when they live on their own. Like a small child, Irene was disconcerted if there was no one in sight. Friends and family had increasingly stepped into the breach, keeping Irene company for chunks of the day, but in between she would ring me persistently at work, sometimes in great distress. This was heartbreaking and stressful for me, as I could do nothing from there. Later, it was easier, as Irene forgot how to make phone calls and by then we had paid help.

I worked four days a week in a demanding job. Being seven years younger than Irene, I was nowhere near retirement age and the thought of leaving my job to 'look after' Irene left me feeling empty. The finances defeated me but I also knew it would do neither of us any good to be together all the time. I know others disagree but this was the right decision for me. In time, I became aware of so many husbands and wives who looked after their partner to the end., That is, to death, or to just a few weeks of being in care. It would have been all-consuming and I knew it would lead to resentment, however much Irene was my love, the centre of my life. I have never felt guilt about this decision as that way madness lies. Instead, I did what I could, which was a lot. My sense that work would be my lifeline turned out to be true.

During the stage when Irene could manage on her own for an hour or so I developed an elaborate rota of people who could come in for short periods. If people can only give an hour or so a week you need an awful lot of people to cover four working days, and I realised it wasn't fair to rely on friends and family. The process of employing people was full of anxiety and stress. Somehow, by hit and miss and asking around, I found a number of connections. People knew other people and, out of a plethora of possibilities, a few likely candidates arrived at our door.

Here are the notes I once wrote for that mixed bag of helpers, some paid, some not. It's strange having people suddenly in your house and responsible for your beloved partner. How to brief them is hard – what do people need to know? The notes give a sense of what Irene was like at this stage:

The aim is to support Irene in what she wants to do, and to provide company. If she wants to do chores, I would see the helper as helping her (e.g. to mow the lawn, clean the car, do the laundry) but I would not see the helper as doing any jobs (e.g. cleaning) for its own sake – i.e. you are there to be with Irene.

There might be times when Irene wants to switch off and not necessarily interact, though she likes to know that there is someone in the house.

Irene does need to be encouraged to eat and drink. There is an additional fridge and freezer in the front porch.

She doesn't take any tablets except at night (one of each of the two packets on her bedside table – Aricept and Sertraline).

Irene enjoys:

Watching the news. News 24 is on all the time on channel 80 using the digi-box. You need to switch on for Irene.

DVD and video come through on ext 2. One of the scart leads is dodgy so if you can't get reception push the scart leads in firmly.

Watching films: Film on Four is through the digi-box.

Watching sport – though we don't have any of the sports channels, if a football or cricket match is on, she'll happily watch.

Going out for coffee.

Walking – lots of walks from the house; OS maps in the dining room. Looking at paintings in galleries.

Writing Amnesty International letters (together). Reading the papers (delivered every day, as is the milk).

Reading her books (may need help finding what she wants to read e.g. in charity shops).

Irene finds difficult:

Handling money especially coins – can't really understand money now; doesn't understand chip and pin if using card in a shop; she can get money from cash machine ok.

Direction finding – best not to let her out of your sight e.g. if in a café, just keep an eye out if she goes to the loo as she might not always see her way back to the table, etc.

Losing things – often cannot locate e.g. her purse; cannot locate the orthotics she wears in her shoes (usually in last pair she had on!); keys (there should be two sets of keys in the kitchen (one set currently lost – I haven't had time to replace); is also a set of keys in the peg bag in the porch overlooking the garden, and next door has a set too.

Keep an eye out that she doesn't leave things, e.g. in cafes or pubs. If something can be left somewhere, Irene is likely to leave it!

Allow plenty of time for her to do things, e.g. getting ready to go out.

Discreetly – If going out check that all the taps are turned off – she sometimes leaves the tap on esp. in the little bathroom. Check doors are locked e.g. door to the garden; garage door. Check periodically that taps aren't left on even if you're staying in, and also stove, iron etc.

 Road safety – don't assume that she can cross roads safely etc; her road sense has gone awry. She does cross roads on her own but just keep an eye out.

If you are held up, ring her as she likes people to be prompt!

If Irene is getting upset, e.g. in the car, pull over, slow the situation down, make sure she feels listened to. Let her let off steam. Step back.

Irene, of course, initially didn't realise she needed help and it was impossible to explain to her why these people were suddenly in our home. She knew our friends and family and could understand their arrival as ordinary social visits. But once I had to employ people it was harder to explain their presence. A lesbian couple came along – I forget who recommended them – and they seemed very good, trustworthy people. They were hoping to work in the dementia field and wanted experience. (You'll get that, I thought.) Because of that, she suggested they be paid as one, in a kind of 'buy one, get one free' deal. Great, £9 an hour instead of £18 was fine by me.

I asked helpers to write the day's happenings in a book so that I would know what had occurred, as Irene would be unable to tell me. These are snippets from what my BOGOF pair wrote from their six stints (on non-consecutive days) before they admitted defeat:

4 September 2006… later we all had a tea and played some table tennis. Irene seemed in good humour. Chatty and full of beans.

11 September 2006   Arrived a little late – rang Irene to let her know, however she didn't understand who I was … when we arrived it was clear she was very agitated and unsettled. Anyway we all went into town to leave her prescription request. Driving there she was fine. However when we were walking into the town centre area it became clear that she was upset we were there. She kept trying to get rid of us, saying, 'You go into this shop and I'll see you later'. She kept storming off and trying to shake us off, to which we still followed her but in a discreet way so she didn't feel so threatened.

To cut a long story short, there's another page and a half of Irene trying to shake them off and they followed her to the bank, Oxfam, a few other places. Then they suggested they all went home. After lunch and a nap, Irene realized she didn't have the greetings cards she'd bought, so they all went back into town and found the cards in the last shop they'd been in…

12 September 2006   A very good day, Irene was chirpy. C and Irene chopped the plums, I washed them and they were stewed and left on the cooker for freezing. We sat and chatted, had a coffee… went to the Garden Centre for lunch…

There follows a long list of all the things Irene ate, and 'overall Irene was much more settled and chatty and funny today'.

14 September 2006   Irene bit upset as Rach's train hadn't turned up so she was worried about Rach getting to London. Rach rang which reassured Irene and we chatted about how bad the trains are. Chatted over tea and then looked at holiday photos, then went for a walk...

26 September 2006   Arrived 10.30. Lorraine [another helper] was already here. When we came into the house it was clear that Irene was distressed and upset. She kept wandering off and sitting alone in other rooms. However after Lorraine left, she picked up her spirits. Irene was her jolly self. There was a list of what they did, including going to the farm shop. Irene bought a lot. They went to the pub for a beer (Irene enjoyed that), a walk by the river, and Irene was settled and happy when we left.

They decided that Irene's behaviour was too much for them and, on what was to be their final day, they describe a day that wasn't untypical of when I was with Irene. It captures what it's like looking after someone in this stage of dementia:

2 October 2006   Had a good start. Got ready to go to the post office. Got sorted and all went to the post office. The staff member got a little impatient. I supervised and we got all the post done. Irene then bought a birthday card for Pippa. Again a little confusion, Irene got upset as she thought she didn't do the posting. We got it all straightened out and off we went to find Pippa's house. [Pippa lives in the same street where we used to live and we have been there many times.] We got to the correct street, but Irene couldn't find the house and when we tried to assist her, she got more agitated. I don't think she signed the card either. When we left, C asked Irene what she wanted to do next. Irene said she didn't care. So we suggested going home and maybe stopping at the farm shop and getting some lunch. However before we got there, as we were driving past a pet food shop, Irene said, 'They make chocolate things in there'. C just said 'Oh, do they make chocolate there?' Then Irene got upset as she wasn't wearing her rings, and started looking for them. I said that maybe they are back at home. And with that she got angry, shouting at me. I didn't say anything more, hoping she would relax and feel better.

We drove on towards home and suddenly Irene shouted that nobody listens, and why didn't we stop for chocolate. C said she didn't realise she wanted to stop and said sorry and asked if Irene wanted us to turn round and go back. With that Irene got really upset. She screamed and started throwing her arms around, banging her fists on the dashboard, shouting for us to stop the car. C said, 'Irene, we are nearly home and we can sort things out over a cuppa'. And then Irene kept shouting and opened the door while the car was moving. Eventually Irene settled but sadly she sobbed all the way home. We were unsure how to manage the whole situation. C made herself scarce by staying in the front room. I made tea and talked to Irene. Irene took her tea up to her room but came down after a few minutes and phoned you. After a while I talked to Irene and explained it was a misunderstanding. C didn't mean to upset her. So I got us all agreeing to go to the farm shop and go for a pub lunch. We went down but the pub lunches were still off as the cook had broken her arm. I bought bread, cheese and eggs. We came home and I made an omelet. We then went in and watched some TV. Left at 2.30 as Irene seemed sleepy and C felt she was making Irene uncomfortable.

It feels so painful now, reading this and knowing that Irene was so unhappy and – what? Frightened? Such behaviour was not unusual that year but I kept no record of it for I was too busy during my three days and seven evenings as a carer, plus four days at my job. I had little time for writing, little time for anything other than getting by.

This wasn't the only time she opened the door of a moving car, not the only time she stormed out of a shop or restaurant, or got angry because she felt no one was taking her seriously. She did it with me too. Once we set off for the Lake District, that special place where Irene was brought up and where we'd had so many happy times. We knew the way blindfolded. But…Irene forced me to stop seven times, insisting we were going the wrong way. She tried to get out of the car, banging her fists; once stationary, she stormed off down the busy highway. I would cajole her back in, set off, try again, double back. I came home twice, and once drove for miles along what I knew was the wrong way, but it kept her happy. We never made it to the Lake District that day – there is symbolism in not being able to get to the place that was so special for us. A kind of madness takes over. You do anything to keep the peace – hold your breath, hope for the demented, crazy minutes to pass into something more recognisable.

These are awful dark days in the dementia story; I can't really encapsulate all the things that happened, the many crises and much heartbreak in the years at home. Now it's a blur of days, and what's left is the pain of wondering how much Irene was conscious of what was happening. I cannot bear to think that she was so unhappy; I cannot, ever, understand what it was like for her. Perhaps the worst (though not the most dramatic or dangerous) day was the time we were sitting on our patio in the sunshine. Irene was upset, knew she was slipping: 'I don't know who I am any more. Please help me.' I cannot think of it even now, years later, without breaking down in tears. It was the most desperate, heart-rending thing I've ever heard. I hugged her, held her, trying to help her keep the threads together but it was perhaps the saddest day of my life. And I have no idea whether it was her worst day because the cruellest thing is that I had no idea, no way of imagining, what it was like for her. And she – she tried to shrug it off too, pull herself together, lest that momentary despair lead to a tidal wave that would sweep us both off our feet.

I was Irene's main helper but I needed amazingly patient, kind people who could cope with Irene's sweet nature and hilarity suddenly turning into fury and frustration. To my utter relief and after weeks of worry, two wonderful women stepped up.

After much asking around I found Chrissie, by her own admission an aging hippy, artist and carer, who was so right it was unbelievable, and with whom Irene felt pretty much instantly comfortable. I thought I had been sent an angel. With her smile, she even looked like one. And there was my niece Emma. As family, she knew Irene and Irene knew her, and as a young mum she needed flexible work and cash. With a lot of other people doing a few hours, it worked – at least for a while. In March 2007, a couple of agencies that gave carers respite also came on board, which enabled me to go to my stress-busting yoga class each week. Eventually, after a lengthy process, we got direct payments from social services to help with the costs.

Looking back, I realise what a strain all this organising was. You're in the middle of a tidal surge so you just keep swimming as hard as you can and keep your head above water. Life was totally bound up with coping with Irene's illness, and I can understand why some partners find it easier to give up everything else and do it full time. Slipping day by day from being a partner to being a carer is gut-wrenchingly awful. Furthermore, as the disease wallops a younger person so much harder, by the time you've set up one system of help care needs have already changed. Anticipating what you might need even a few months ahead is impossible. Knowing that nothing is forever kept me going: time passes, hard times fade. I knew that when ours did I would take myself off to the Arctic, as if the white cold of the Polar Regions could cauterize something. I realise too that all those little incidents fitted together. When we went on holiday, maybe on a boat, and Irene still hadn't learned by the end of the week what the layout was and would have to search afresh, say, for the fridge, each time she needed it and then progressively forgot where things went in our own kitchen…

It's easier to talk about memory, much harder to talk about her behaviour. in a café she'd send a coffee back because it was 'too hot', or she'd flee from a restaurant and refuse to come back in, her meal going cold and the waiters pretending not to notice a commotion going on. If there with friends, we'd be talking amongst ourselves about who should go and remonstrate with Irene, or if Irene and I were on our own I'd plead with her not to make a scene. Not that I minded people seeing, rather I just wanted us to relax and enjoy the time.

There were happy times too. We had a big celebration for our 25th anniversary in the autumn of 2005 and we had our civil partnership in February 2006, getting in on the first wave after it became legal. We'd bought a ring for Irene a couple of weeks before, in a little jewellery shop in the Picos Mountains in northern Spain where we were holidaying. We were served by a tiny Spanish woman, who probably would have thrown us out if she'd known it was for a civil partnership. Irene had one of the conversations with her that people either picked up on as not being quite normal or thought was a great lark. Our señora fell into the latter group, while I stood by nervously, not sure if it was one of those occasions when things would get out of hand.

We had arranged the civil ceremony for the last session on a Friday afternoon and had told only a couple of friends. It snowballed and we had about forty people at the registry office. Everyone knew Irene had Alzheimer's.

Everyone knew there was an urgency about it. There wasn't a dry eye in the house as we exchanged vows. Afterwards we went to a local hotel and took over their very large bar. A few other quiet drinkers grew puzzled and then looked alarmed when they realised the happy occasion was actually a civil partnership. Irene's brother said a few words (even though we'd said no speeches) and he paid for champagne. We then went to an Indian restaurant with our close family. Irene was on cloud nine, loving every minute. We just made it – we needed a change to our wills and other documents to be signed by someone in full possession of their faculties. Irene wasn't really in full possession by any means, but she was happy with it all and would not have wanted it any other way.

We carried on walking as we had always done and attempted, in sections, to walk from Land's End to John o' Groats. We got as far as Helmsdale, 50-odd miles short in Scotland, and had got as far as Somerset in the southerly direction. We did Devon in the spring of 2006 but it left me so nervously exhausted, trying to coax Irene along and anticipate her behaviour, that I knew the game was up. We would either never finish it or I would do it alone. Well, it didn't matter so much in the scheme of things. We had an extraordinary number of holidays: to France to see the grave of my great uncle again; to Prague; a week in the Italian lakes; to Holland, where we stayed with friends; a week in Denmark with Irene's brother and his wife; and a week near Capri.

We had quiet times at home. Irene was happiest doing art work, with me or Chrissie or Emma. I asked a friend who is a film maker to make a short film of us in the garden. I wanted something, for me. In it she talks and laughs, caught forever as she was then. The most poignant part for me is when she talks about her previous amateur dramatics, the fun she had, and then says, as if it's news to the listener: 'I couldn't do it now, no, I couldn't do it now'.

Diary of a Secret Social Services User

During these years I had increasingly to engage with social services and health services to get the right help for both of us. This piece, about that process, was originally written for the Alzheimer's Society newsletter. The Alzheimer's Society (bless them!) realised they needed to embrace the 21st century diversity agenda so they had set up an LGBT project which included a helpline staffed by members of the LGBT community. I was asked to write a couple of pieces for the newsletter by Roger, a lovely guy on the helpline, who proved to be such a joy. His own partner of 30 years had also developed Alzheimer's and he provided advice and support in a way that a professional could not have done. I don't know how typical were my experiences with social services. Some of our problems were caused by the fact that we lived in a peculiar little pocket of the countryside with boundaries co-terminus with nothing very much. Our postcode looked fictional, our political constituency gerrymandered. These facts didn't matter greatly but what did come to matter was that because we'd kept our GP when we'd moved house, our health care and our social care came under two different counties. That apart, my encounter with bureaucracy and statutory services reads like the nightmare that it was:

April 2006 Application form for Disability Living Allowance (DLA) arrives. Well, not a form, more like a booklet. Pages and pages. Remind myself I have a PhD. I can do this.

May 2006 Humongous form finally goes off, after being filled in where appropriate by our Community Psychiatric Nurse (CPN). She says we need to get into the social care system and will set this up. A few months go by...

August 2006 Meet nice social worker, though she talks a lot and I have to interrupt to ask her what I need to know. She's with the Younger People with Dementia Team. First a visit to us at home, then with me on my own at the Alzheimer's Society HQ to fill in a needs assessment form – to assess Irene's needs so we can apply for direct payments which is where the state will pay us and we will then pay carers selected by us rather than social services carers coming in. She says I will need to have another interview for a financial assessment.

September 2006   Notice large and unexpected amount deposited in our current account. Could it be the DLA? The D could stand in for 'Delayed' but at least it's backdated for the five months it's taken for it to be processed. Fairly good news re the level they have put us on – except that in the intervening months Irene's disease has worsened so now we would probably qualify for a higher rate, but I can't face reapplying just yet…

October 2006   Nice social worker phones, embarrassed. Er, actually as we don't live in County X we are not eligible to proceed, but instead have to start the whole process again with our own social services team, in County Y. Very sorry etc etc and our CPN will contact County Y. So we are back to where we were two months ago.

Meanwhile, Irene has rejected the outreach worker from the Alzheimer's Society, two care workers I engaged myself have decided they can't deal with Irene's behaviour and have given a day's notice while a third gets a full-time job. Luckily, I find Chrissie who, after a slightly rocky start, settles in and covers two days a week. Irene loves her. I am relying on her and a rota of friends, forking out about double what the DLA covers.

We continue with monthly visits from our wonderful CPN interspersed with visits from another female consultant. The crisis management of the last few months begins to settle down, though it's all still a roller coaster.

November 2006   Discuss the conundrum caused by geography with our CPN. I don't want to lose our health care in County X with its greater provision and still can't face starting again with another team. Neither would this help Irene. But we definitely can't access social care in County X and County Y so far hasn't responded to CPN's overtures.

January 2007   Social worker from county Y pops up and a meeting is arranged at our house. We start again at the point we were at five months ago with previous social worker. This one seems perplexed and unnerved by Irene and a tricky situation is rescued by the student psychiatric nurse our CPN has brought with her, who whisks her away to Irene's makeshift art room (our dining room) to inspect her latest art work. Another meeting is arranged so we can discuss Irene's case.

February 2007   I take a friend to said meeting and we forget it's school half term so we get there quickly through light traffic, arriving half an hour early. Social worker arrives half an hour late as she gets lost (well, we are in a different county after all). Bombshell – as we are in County X for our health care but in county Y for social care, and as the day centre in County X is run by social services and in county Y by health services, we can't access either... My algebra fails me at this point but I know it adds up to an injustice. CPN and social worker look grave and realise that they will actually have to sort out a co-operative arrangement. Friend and I emerge after several hours feeling we need a pick-me-up but instead having to get to work.

March 2007   Meet with social worker, who seems more at ease in her home office. Long interview, which is a carer's assessment. I have already filled in a questionnaire where I just ticked Yes to everything. 'Ooh,' she says, 'it does look like your caring role affects your life.' (Doh!) Questions are somewhat blunt: e.g. 'Does your caring role affect your emotional and/or physical health?' Er, well, let me think about that for a pica-second. In our early fifties I'm losing the person I've spent half my life with and whom I want to spend the rest of it with, we've lost our lovely retirement together and I am heartbroken – does that do for the emotional bit? And I've had cancer, wake every two hours in the night and always feel tired. Is that OK for the physical bit? About 20 other questions in a similar vein. We decide to put down a sum for the counselling paid for by me twice a month for the last year-and-a-half – expensive, but it's what keeps me sane enough to fulfil the caring role which otherwise the state would have to take on. Lots of other suggestions too re organisations which offer sitters, respite, etc, but it's a bewildering scene of charities, agencies, people to contact, forms to send off for. I'm told that we can apply for a Council Tax rebate of up to half the amount, which in our case amounts to about a thousand pounds. Wonder why no one told me that before? Feel like I need a few days off work and away from my caring role to sort all this out.

Social worker will ask her manager (on leave at present) if County Y will pay for Irene to attend the day centre in County X, who have already agreed as long as County Y pays up. County X warns that there's waiting list though…

Later in March   Meet with financial assessor who has sent a long list of the paperwork she needs to see. Broken heart sinks. Think about mess of our filing system. (Not much time left to keep files in order when you look after a person with dementia.) Remind myself I'm in a responsible job. I can do this. Surprise myself at how much of it I manage to conjure up but still fall at certain hurdles: e.g. our last four electricity bills, water bills… Surprise myself at how upset I feel about her suggestion of setting up a separate bank account for Irene and separating out some items. Jumbling of our finances has always been a sign of commitment for me and has always worked.

Even later in March   Social worker phones to say that county Y will pay for the day centre and is processing the application for direct payments. (By now I've been paying out for carers since September 2006 so that I can carry on going to work four days a week.) Feels like two steps forward… so what's the step back? Ah well, there's a clause she's just noticed which says that the person in receipt of direct payments (i.e. Irene) has to be able to manage the administration at the point where the direct payments start, i.e. to open a bank account, recruit and pay the carers, etc. I point out that if Irene was compos mentis she wouldn't be needing carers and direct payments… It appears that as I have enduring power of attorney, Irene might not be able to receive direct payments… I suggest that this is discriminating against people with dementia. She asks me whether, when we started this process, now eight months ago, Irene would have been able at that point to understand and carry out the process. Ah, I think for another pica-second, the right answer is Yes, so I say, 'Yes'… Even though the true answer is No… She says she will go away and find out more from an expert. I wonder who that might be. I am left astounded. Direct payment seems ideal for us and I can't believe this latest obstacle. Various people are on leave, including our CPN. It's April soon, a year since I filled in the application for DLA to start the process of getting some financial help with caring. I wonder how people in less fortunate financial situations than we are manage.

Looking back on this now, it still feels like a nightmare, and that's with all the considerable personal and external resources I had at my disposal. I had a lot of help from the Alzheimer's Society. A wonderful woman came out to see me at work and talked things through. Her best advice was to keep it all simple. She also told me to be assertive, for example when our GP had told me to tell Irene that she could no longer drive. That was preposterous she said, and I should not have to be the one to tell Irene anything negative. It was someone else's job. It was certainly true that she should not have been driving, a huge marker in the dementia journey. Irene was both relieved and outraged. I still have dreams where Irene is at the wheel of a car. I know that she shouldn't be driving but somehow a lapse of (my) concentration means that she is.

That GP suddenly left the surgery and we felt temporarily abandoned. As it turned out, we came under an even better (woman) GP who was incredibly kind and supportive. Our CPN carried on being amazing, and we carried on having home visits, sometimes with the psychiatric consultant, an equally capable and caring woman who accompanied her. Irene really liked them both.

The Alzheimer's Society's LGBT project wound up after two years, but the other really positive outcome was that I made contact with the only other woman I've found who was in my position, with her partner in a further stage of dementia than Irene. The problem was she lived in New Zealand. Anyway, we emailed and became a source of some comfort to each other.

The second year of the secret diary shows it wasn't as frustrating, but it does show Irene's inevitable decline:

Year 2 of the diary of a secret social services user

March 2007   I go abroad with my work, leaving an elaborate rota of people in charge. Irene misplaces her wallet at a friend's house in the Lake District and later cannot find it. Friends root through our files etc. at home to find out what to cancel etc. as Irene hasn't a clue. One night Irene leaves the bathroom tap running, with (unusually) the plug in. Pauline has a flooded kitchen floor to deal with at 3 a.m. one morning. Apart from this, no major mishaps... Wallet turns up a few days after my return.

April 2007   Irene and I are invited to go to the day centre at the Alzheimer's Society to see if Irene likes it. We go in just as everyone is assembled and doing a word search game as a warm-up for the day. Irene doesn't have a clue what's going on and neither, it seems, do quite a few of the other users and I wonder what the point of this game is. I resist trying to help out by suggesting a few words and the whole thing reminds me of the word puzzle my mother used to do in her evening paper every day, to ward off dementia. We have a tour of the premises and I get the impression Irene thinks she might be being enrolled as a new helper. A few days later she has the chance to try out a morning there. Irene isn't sure she wants to go. 'There were some funny people there,' she says. My sister Penny and niece Emma take her. Both are in tears leaving her and nearly decide not to. I make the mistake of someone else picking her up (I'm at work), which confuses Irene.

CPN rings that afternoon to say she's not sure this will work – I'd already realised that, from Irene's reaction. Irene's poor hearing is one factor but also it's just not right and Irene can't engage with it all. It's OK – whatever is right for her is what we need. All that bargaining on access…Well, too bad.

May 2007   We have a holiday in Italy. Irene really wanted to go, after the success of Italy in October 2006. But this is a disaster. We should not be on our own; my sister Mary can be with us for half the time but once she leaves we lock horns in a peculiar way. For example, after dropping Mary at the airport, I face a two or three-hour drive back to our villa. Irene insists we stop for a meal – we'd just had a break at the airport and I wanted to get a move on. I explain this, but each and every restaurant we pass – most of them closed as it's too early in Italy for them to be open – Irene insists we stop. I eventually lose it. Irene says, with great insight, 'I think we're OK when we have someone else with us.' It's too much for me to entertain Irene. We have one peaceful afternoon, with Irene painting and me sitting quietly with her. But mainly it's too hard and I am lonely, out of sorts, stressed.

June 2007   Life continues with a rota of helpers to be with Irene 24/7 except for the very occasional half hour when there's a gap. One day, with no warning, £6,500 turns up in the bank account I've opened to receive direct payments. I go to meet the Independent Living Scheme, a charity which helps people administer direct payments. They are a godsend. My brain seems unable to function around this, all efficiency disappearing under the emotional toll that this task is wreaking. I am absolutely hopeless at getting the payments right; I don't understand how I can be so bad at this – I've got a responsible job but I guess it doesn't include accountancy.

Part Two: Going into Care

Falling Through the Ice

In 29 August 2007 Irene was admitted to an acute psychiatric hospital. It turned out to be her last day at home, the day she 'went into care'. It is one of those few dates in your life story against which you measure everything as either coming before or after it, like 9/11. I wrote about it at the time, just to try to capture it: you think you will remember, but even something you think will be seared into your memory gets jumbled with time. Some of what follows is based on those jottings.

Two weeks previously we had been cycling in Holland, albeit with the safety net of several friends and family. Two weeks before that we had been canoeing on the river in our new inflatable canoe and Irene had loved it, the peace and quiet of the river, floating along, watching swans preening in the summer's evening light. It was one of those special moments of calm that it was still possible to share with Irene, as of old.

But there had also been an escalation of more dramatic moments.

We'd had a disastrous foray north to Harris, an island too far, in July 2007. We'd gone to see a friend as part of her sixtieth birthday celebrations. On the way back, we'd called in at Irene's brother's. By now, I could take no more, after two weeks of being with Irene and her, at times, appalling behaviour. I did not realise then that Irene had phases where she didn't know who I was, which meant she felt she was driving in a strange car with a strange person in a landscape she didn't recognise. No wonder she panicked or threw a wobbly, shouted at me or tried to get away. It was stormy, to say the least. The most dangerous moment was when she grabbed the steering wheel when I was doing 70 mph in the middle lane of the motorway. I think she even shocked herself at that one. As we pulled away from her brother's to drive south, she turned to me and said, 'I don't know why I didn't recognise you – maybe it's because I haven't seen you for a few months.' So she knew enough to know that she didn't know – the worst of all confusions.

Then – a bombshell. Chrissie resigned, feeling she was now out of her depth. She had become really fond of Irene so it was a big step for her too. My other carefully constructed care plans were also unravelling.

Now, rather than the odd day of furious behaviour, upset and exhaustion fuelled by Irene's paranoia, there were whole weeks of it. 'I WANT YOU TO CALL THE POLICE!' Irene was seeing me as someone malign and out to get her. 'THIS IS NOT MY HOUSE!' or, alternatively, 'THIS IS MY HOUSE – GET OUT!' she shouted. In the middle of August, Irene furiously threw me out of the house early one morning as she thought she had an intruder. (She had locked me out the week before too.) Fortunately, Jean, one of Irene's best friends, was due to arrive with another old university pal to take Irene away for a few days and give me a break. They found me miserably hanging around on the street corner. Before long, Irene wanted to come home and, on their return, her behaviour was so erratic that Jean felt she needed to stay. She left on Sunday.

On Tuesday we had the scheduled visit from our psychiatrist, who recommended that Irene go into hospital to get her medication sorted out. How long for? I kept asking, to which she replied, 'A few weeks, two or three?' Irene started to pack her own bag before the doctor had even left the house. She clearly wanted to be off, she wanted help. But I was in some sort of panic and scared of the consequences of Irene leaving home for any length of time (and so forgetting it forever), so I prevaricated. I saw the short periods of calm as evidence that Irene really wasn't too bad. I wasn't seeing the bizarre behaviour, the fear, confusion and deterioration that so plainly showed that Irene had entered another new phase. I was incapable of making a decision about what action to take, whether to let Irene go into hospital or to stay at home, and I let go the bed which had been arranged and which was available to us only for the next 24 hours. Our CPN was due to call the next afternoon and I decided I would do whatever she recommended. She said it was absolutely clear – it was time for Irene to be in hospital.

Wednesday 29 August. Just before we left the house, Irene and I were suddenly alone together in the living room in a little oasis of calm after all the comings and goings and all of the drama. We stood close to one another, and she turned to me and said, 'It's OK Rach, it won't be for long and we'll always have each other.' Just seconds before, she didn't seem to even know who I was. After all the upset, nervous tension and despair of the previous weeks and days, here she was saying something that was so full of love and care and insight that it still takes my breath away. It still astounds me when I think of it, that she was comforting me.

I was told I had to drive Irene to the city centre hospital myself. I called my sister, who lived only nine miles away, and she rushed over. She sat in the back of the car with Irene as I drove. She had both of us to worry about, me blinded with tears and Irene now extremely agitated and trying to get out of the car, no longer thinking she was on a journey to safety. We were expected, and one of those young doctors – who looks like a college kid and makes you feel old – made an assessment. He was competent and kind, and gave Irene something to read on a clipboard. She put ticks against whatever was written there, as if she was marking his school work. She did it so authentically, so professionally, that the doctor had to smile, and so did we. We then sat on Irene's bed, not sure what to do next. Leaving her at the hospital was devastating beyond words, and Irene herself kept saying to the admissions doctor: 'Well, thank you very much but we have to be going now,' picking up her little bag and making for the door.

I returned the next morning just as the consultant was about to see Irene. He was a straightforward young man, with a trendily bald head. I liked him. Irene sat in the consultation with us, but she was very distressed and kept repeating loudly, 'I HAVE DONE NOTHING WRONG!', evidently believing that she had been sent away to be punished. My poor love. I had to keep it together to talk to the consultant. I couldn't comfort her. Torture. He had clearly made a quick assessment based on experience and could see that Irene was not out of place on an acute ward, but he stunned me by saying that getting the medication right was going to take two or three months rather than two or three weeks. I asked him to give it to me straight and he said it was unlikely that Irene would go home again after this.

I thought she was being admitted for two to three weeks to get her medication sorted out. Bang! It dawned on me that the decision I'd been dreading making, one that floated hazily on a distant horizon, had now

41

been made. Irene was admitted and it looked like she might never come home again. This massive hurdle was suddenly behind me. Without my noticing, we'd cleared it. The unbearable thought of Irene in care was no longer in front of me but behind, and all I could do for the moment was to look over my shoulder to try to puzzle out how it had actually happened.

I asked the consultant how it was possible to deteriorate this quickly. He pulled out a handy analogy: it's like walking on thin ice and the ice is getting thinner and thinner but you don't especially notice this…until suddenly you fall through that ice and your world is suddenly so, so different. The feeling of being up in the air, albeit on a slippery surface, is utterly different from floundering in the cold, dark and wet of a frozen lake from which you cannot possibly extricate yourself unaided. He said that the cracks had been harder to see because Irene had started with a high IQ and I had put in place such a good system of care at home. This all made sense. It's like blowing up a bridge – it's either totally there or totally gone. Something for Irene was totally gone. The GP's assessment of three or four years in the end turned out to be two-and-a-half.

It was blindingly obvious to everyone except me that admitting Irene was the right decision. I thought we could surely have still managed at home, that she didn't really need this; not now, not yet. After a whole week of going over and over the necessity of it with everyone and anyone, I then had another week of rolling waves of relief, some of the stress lifting, and of being extraordinarily tired. I'd had no time at all off work during Irene's decline to this point – somehow I'd kept the show on the road, with the help of very understanding colleagues. Now I could look back and realise that I had seen the cracks opening up; we'd had those terrible times of really difficult behaviour but somehow I had just managed. Your sense of what's normal and what's a crisis becomes completely distorted when you live with someone with Alzheimer's. Although I had held my breath, carried on doing the things which Irene herself wanted to do, tried to keep a quality of life, it had been falling apart. Friends and relatives were amazed at what we did still manage to achieve. But it couldn't go on. We were bound to fall through the ice sooner or later.

That first night that Irene was in hospital I understood what Shakespeare meant by being mad with grief. It's a feeling I never want to experience again. All I can say is that it really is everything you think 'madness' means, and more. You lose your mind.

Nevertheless, I got into some sort of routine and went from looking after Irene's needs 24/7 to just visiting her. The hospital was near my workplace, so I went every weekday. Irene was different each time. Some days she was hardly even aware of me. One day she put her arms round me and said, 'I love you.' Then she asked how long she would have to be there, adding 'We have a lovely home.' I took her outside when I could, and we would walk around the block. She was well-behaved and had lost the need to be furious. This was welcome but at the same time sad, as the fight had gone from her. Better for her, no doubt, but oh, the desperate awfulness of leaving her in that place!

Initially she was on an admission ward, which was pretty benign and the other patients took to her, helping her out. Then she was moved to the dementia ward which I'm sure wasn't like a Dickensian bedlam but it didn't feel far off. Just a 21st-century reincarnation of it. I found it grim, a T-shape of corridor with bedrooms off it. It felt like a prison. She deteriorated further as the creeping institutionalisation set in and she moved further from the one-to-one care at home. Three weeks in, I began to allow myself to grieve for my partner in a way I hadn't been able to while she was at home. She was still there, but not the person she was, a partner both lost but present. Looking back, that time still feels like one of the worst; helpers, friends, and service providers think that's when it's all over and the carer/partner, will feel relieved.

In reality, it's just the start of another kind of trauma. Different demands, different emotions – and for me it was when the real grieving began.

Irene was in the acute psychiatric hospital from 29 August to 5 November. She was moved from there to an NHS-run community home, a kind of half-way house and a huge improvement, to await assessments and a decision as to what to do next.

Letters to Irene

In October 2007 I started to write letters to Irene. She would never read them but it made me feel better. I had seen her every day in the acute hospital and I needed a break; I had a work trip due and, rather hesitantly, I went. It felt terrible – mainly guilt but also worry –yet Irene was where she had to be, and I needed some respite.

Letter to Irene on our 27th anniversary, 22 October 2007

Dear Part of My Heart,

I miss you with all that I have. The other day you didn't know who I was but today you did. You said my name and you said, 'I love you'. I was too choked with tears to say anything, and anyway you didn't have your hearing aids in so you wouldn't have heard me. You were not in the mood for hearing anyway, but for talking. You chattered away quite happily and laughed a lot though I didn't know what you were saying. It made sense to you, which is the important thing, and you seemed happy.

It has been so hard seeing you in these days since I got back from being away. Hard to reintegrate into what our lives have become. I miss you and I feel lonely here on my own. I went today to see the place where I hope you will go to live. It's nice and I liked the owner who seemed to have such a respect for people with dementia. I think you will like it and be happy there. I feel a bit upset that I missed a vacancy that came up only last week and I wondered if I'd been here we could have taken it. But they might not have released you from the hospital yet and maybe I just have to accept that what will be will be. I hope you don't have to wait too many months to get in there. There are some people as young as you, some women that seem like you and that you would get on with. It has a nice garden and trees to look at.

I hope it works out. I realise now that we need to get you out of the hospital and into a more social environment and a more normal place. I won't feel settled until it happens.

I love you. I'm crying now, have been since I got back. Who would have thought we'd spend our 27th anniversary like this? At least you connected with me today. Love you to the end. Can't say any more just now, can't see the keyboard for tears.

23 October

Dear Irene,

You didn't seem to know me today. I forgot to say yesterday that when I was in the home where I hope you will go. Janet, the owner, showed us around and she asked me for a penny so she could open someone's bedroom for us to have a look. The doors have some kind of lock that you can open with a coin if no key is around. Anyway, she gave me back the penny and I dropped it. We couldn't find it and I thought, good, maybe that means you will go there if the penny wants to stay. Then Janet found it, and gave it to me. I decided to leave it there in a hiding place but as we went around couldn't decide where to put it. I thought about chucking it under a tree in the garden, somewhere it couldn't be found, but then I saw a water feature which had just been built, a sort of raised bed. It had old railway sleepers to make the sides and there was a series of holes which were exactly penny sized, so I shoved it down, face up, about an inch. I don't think anyone could winkle it out. I hope it will stay there and that you will eventually go there.

I am very tired and I cry a lot. I have lost you, my partner, my life.

24 October

Dear Little Person,

I didn't come to see you today. I'm sorry. I want to see you and have missed seeing you but I just felt like I needed a day off and I couldn't rise to it. I will see you tomorrow. I have a lot of time that I'm not sure what to do with; there're no little routines or rituals. No one notices I'm home, so I just make a cup of tea and then wonder what to do next. I haven't been going into the living room. I guess that was where we spent a lot of time. I'm tending to be in the computer room or places where I used to be on my own, rather than where we were together.

I feel like I will have the rest of this year letting myself be a leaky bucket as I want to cry it all out. I can't believe how upset I can be still. Nothing really sparks it off, just thinking of you and what you are like now. The fish are OK. I will get the final batch soon, another bottom feeder to replace the poor one which died. It upsets me to see it on its own without another like it. The tank was in a real mess but I enjoyed getting it all cleaned up again.

I'm sorry I didn't see you today. Wonder whether I should come in now but I'm back home and I am tired. Are you OK? I'm pretty lonely. Love you.

PS I was wondering about wearing your watch. Not sure if it will upset me too much but I might like to wear it and the practical side of me thinks I might as well.

25 October

Dear Giggly Person,

You giggled all the time today and chatted sometimes with words that I could understand. It's better if you lie on the bed as then we can look at each other as your stooped neck means I can't see your face when you are standing. You said, 'I love you' and I was too choked to reply. You did know who I was then, though later you said I was called Wendy. One time you looked at me closely and said, 'You look tired.' I said, 'I am,' and you said, 'Are you?' It was a kind of conversation. We don't have conversations anymore. You would say all sorts of things, some of which was proper words but often not, then laugh like mad. We both laughed in fact and at one point you said, 'Oh stop it!' in fits of giggles, just like we used to. I left you on your bed and I don't think you would have known that I'd gone.

Last night when I couldn't sleep I was wondering about changing the rooms round. I'd quite like to have your study, to sit where you used to sit, be near you – and it always did have the best view. Then the computer room could be a proper spare room, as I'd move the computer into your little study (and still have my big study). All this space! It's our house somehow; you're kind of here. All your stuff, which you won't need any more and I guess at some point I will have to go through it all.

26 October

Dear Irene,

I hope you are OK today. I wasn't in town so I didn't come in to see you. That's twice in a week I've not been in and it feels strange. I think of you alone in there and it is painful. Yes, it feels painful. I don't know if I have the energy to do what I have to, and all I want to do is lie down. Hope you are getting rest too; miss you.

28 October

Dearest,

You were on form today, talking all the time and chuckling every few minutes. You seemed to know who I was though you didn't recognise Mary or Dave [my brother and sister]. It was when you looked at me for a long time without saying anything and then said 'I'd like to go somewhere with you' that I cried. A big tear splashed on your leg. I had to look down for a long time or I would have dissolved completely and I don't know what you would make of that.

There's new woman on the ward called Norma; she is very attractive and looks so young, in her prime. She demanded some keys from [my brother] David and I was annoyed with the nurse Paul, who really was the culprit yet he didn't come over to intervene. It now seems that, apart from the more elderly patients, you have been there longer than anyone else. You haven't I guess, but a lot of other faces have been and gone.

It felt like you were speeding today, all your movements fast. You would shoot off once you had a mind to and I like it better when you are lying on your bed and we can look at each other. Your head and neck are still very bent. I guess they haven't yet got the medication right, as this speeding isn't natural. It's been two months now. One of the things that's hard is that you left for a short time, or so we thought, yet this is forever, and you had no time to say goodbye to the house or take the things that you would have liked. On that day, 29 August, we had a few minutes together in the living room and for a few seconds you seemed completely lucid and knew what was happening. You hugged me and said, 'It's OK, it will only be for a while'. You knew that I needed consoling, you knew you were leaving. That was amazing and with hindsight perhaps one of the most profound few minutes of my life, and of our life together.

29 October

Dear Mrs Chuckles,

The new patient, Norma, reminded me of you a few months ago, urgently asking me to call the police, and then later doing a dance quite happily. Remember when you first went there, there was a tea dance on your second day and we danced together. Seems an age ago. We laughed today and I fed you your meal, plus a whole punnet of chopped fruit which you seemed to like a lot. The doctor said the brain scan didn't show any damage other than the AD and they are still waiting for the X-ray results for your poor neck. I said maybe it's time to get you out of there and to the half-way community care home. Is that the right thing? I wish you could tell me. I wish we could communicate properly. The doctor asked if I talked about things, reminded you of our life and so on. I don't – I think I would crack up and it always feels cruel to remind you of another life, that life we had long ago. Anyway, you don't seem to respond to my words, or any conversation. You suddenly seem to have lost the ability to take in words. I wonder what you know, what you think, what you are saying to yourself. You mentioned your mother today and Gordon but I'm not sure you knew me.

2 November

The other day when I got off the train there was a car waiting to pick someone up and for an instant I thought how lovely if it was you, like you used to pick me up to save me walking up the hill. Hard to think I'll never have anyone to do that and that there won't be anyone in the house when I get home, the fire lit.

Anyway, yesterday when I saw you we had some quality time, you lying on the bed and me sitting with you. That point where you looked at me hard for a few minutes and then said, 'I think you're going to cry,' and you seemed to know who I was and what was happening, doing that thing which often used to happen where we echoed each other exactly and became one being. Us as a couple rather than two separate people, so that we weren't sure which one had spoken, and we knew that the other could see what was going on in the other's mind. And I did think I was going to cry, that was exactly what was in my mind as we had a connecting for a few seconds which was so real and so sad, a glimpse of a past which has gone, like seeing something very far away through clouds parting.

I am finding it hard to be on the ward. I don't mind the guy who takes all his clothes off or the other things you see and expect when people are this ill. No, it's to do with the new people there, the ones who are young and very disturbed. Norma is articulate and knows there are huge conspiracies against her, people coming to murder her. The black nurse who is trying to poison her. It reminds me of you a few months ago, and I feel a huge sense of sadness knowing that this bright, pert woman is going to be lost in a few months' time. I don't want to see a decline all over again. I can't be a witness again. Sometimes she does a little dance and a song and I bet like you, she used to entertain people.

I'm sorry we didn't get to cut your hair. I wish your neck were normal. It is hard to see you like this. You are thin and your trousers kept slipping, not helped by the button having come off. You had a kind of nappy on, and I realise that your body, which I used to know so well, is now becoming unknown to me, as I don't enquire about what you are still able to do and what you can't. Norma told a lovely story about how she was seeing her father; a long story where it turned out that it wasn't her father, but the Lord. It was a special moment and meant something to her. Your own monologue punctuated it in just the right places, which was sweet and funny too.

Gordon will be coming at the weekend. I'll see you later today too.

3 November

Dear Special Person,

I thought of lots of things I wanted to tell you and now my mind's gone blank. You know that time when you're lying in bed, awake, but not ready to get up and your mind starts thinking? We had some special moments yesterday, with you saying, 'You are lovely; I love you'. I have done everything I can to get you moved to a nicer place, and that will happen I promise. Maybe Monday or Tuesday. Gordon and I are looking at it today.

Miss you. I'm sort of OK. I'm enjoying more than I thought I would, being on my own. I feel like I'm still with you when I'm on my own rather than having to beam in to other people. And this time is a bonus, when you and I can communicate, I mean in the hospital, when you recognise me and say loving things. I need that. This feels like our Indian Summer. This always was our time of year, autumn sunshine falling on golden leaves, a blue sky and sudden intensity of light which seems to set the world afire.

Wonder how many other people have been through this, losing a great love, a profound love. I will not do a Queen Victoria. Life is too short. And I still have you, for a while yet anyway.

5 November

Dear One,

Haven't seen you over the weekend. I was working in the garden cutting back the ivy hedge and it was so lovely, that autumn sunshine, and I was happy just stopping to stare at things. The garden looks lighter and bigger, the way it always does when we chop the hedges to death. Hope the move happens today. Love you.

Later…

Bonfire night and bangs going off like crazy outside. You'd hate it. Well, the move seems to have gone OK except for them losing your hearing aid, which I'll have to go in search of. It's your better ear too. You don't seem to be that aware of having moved but your new room is much nicer and I feel happier about it. We had one of the best conversations today. Seems to happen when you are lying down and we can see each other. You said, 'Why can you see, see the sea, see the sea, the sea and you can't see me?'

Profound or what? I have been seeing the sea but I can't be with you. You were asking me in your own way why we couldn't live together. You also said how lovely I was and how you loved me, several times. I managed to respond more too, and at one point I lay down and put my head on your chest, and you knew I was crying. You knew. You quivered a bit too but you also laughed a lot, though not as much as usual. The fireworks are whizzing outside. Oh, but I don't miss all the tension, wondering if you were going to be OK or have a strop. I can't go through that again. If I ever fell in love again and they started to get dementia, would I quit and run? Yes, I think I would. Talking to Pauline [Irene's sister-in-law] and she said how amazing I was through all that but now I don't want to think about it, I can't go there – too hard, too painful. What's happening in your mind? What was happening then? What a cruel disease. Good night, sweet dreams with no loud bangs. Love ya.

10 November

Dear Mrs,

Well you are in your new home, albeit a temporary one, and you confounded us yesterday, laughing and singing. You were really pleased to see me, held on to my hands tightly and we sat for a long while holding hands. Then Barbara came in and you knew her too, and we took you outside for a walk. I saw the hairdresser's shop so we went in and hey presto they could do your hair there and then, so we did. A bit of an effort but a short back and sides so now can see your face. You were really on form and were reading words from the magazines in there. Amazing. Barbara and I were laughing. Today you did know me at first but then walked past me in the corridors as if I wasn't anyone special to you. You were singing little tunes and laughing. Gosh I'm tired.

13 November

Dear Irene,

You are singing loudly and without inhibition which is quite funny given you could never sing in tune and that one of your party stories was the one where you'd joined a choir and the leader asked to hear it but without you … You said my name several times last night and also Gordon's and Kirkley Bank [Irene's parents' old house]. I hope you can stay there for the foreseeable future. I have been drinking more red wine but sometimes it gives me a really bad headache, like now… I was startled the other day to think I had only 17 years till I'm 70 and red wine has lots of antioxidants etc. so maybe it will help, but on the other hand these headaches aren't much fun. Think I'd not eaten enough as I wanted to see you and missed meal times. Bye for now.

Later today: I feel lonely tonight. I miss you! I haven't seen you today and I miss you when I don't. Can't see you tomorrow either. What do I do with all your things? Two bikes in the garage. Feel tired; can't deal with too much of people. I'd like just to see you, come home, mooch about, read my book. I don't really want to make an effort. Miss you.

18 November

Dear Irene,

I need to say goodbye and this is me saying goodbye, listening to Schubert's Impromptus, especially the one in G-flat because it's about reconciliation to loss. I can't carry on writing to you as if you really read what I say; what I write is emotionally honest – I mean all that I write – but it's no longer honest because it's not real. You are so far beyond any understanding. You are lost and I have lost you.

That's all I can say because that's all that's left. It's too painful to remember how you were and the reality is that you are only a small speck of what you were. You are a person now who is very ill and very confused, very demented. I don't know how much longer you will survive and I know that the next big thing for me to come to terms with is you dying, because I think you will die sooner rather later. I can no longer fool myself that we have some kind of sunshine in our lives together. Maybe a few specks now and then but really your life is elsewhere and mine is here. The reality is a person wandering corridors in a world of their own, cared for by kind strangers. You are no longer mine but everybody's.

Chrissie talked of a little spark of love glowing in the hospital, which was comforting a couple of months ago but it feels more and more faint, like something that was rather than something that is. The reality is that I have to get used to what you have become. I can't pretend that we still have something when really we haven't. Unless this is real, everything is lost.

Love you forever though.

Review Meeting

My diary records one of the many review meetings that took place during this time when it was being decided what Irene's needs were.

20 December 2007 How are you supposed to react when the medical team tell you that your life partner and soul mate has been found eating her own faeces?

I suspected she was doubly incontinent and the nurse confirmed it by speaking the words. The large nappy she's worn for a while gave me a rather large clue but … doubly incontinent. I knew that's what people with dementia eventually succumbed to but it seems incongruous with Irene's increased awareness of me, her affection and her saying the words 'I love you' and 'All I want is you' and often a jumble of words that actually say it more than anything else could, like today, 'I am you and you are me.'

It seems they need three people to change her and take care of personal hygiene, as she can be resistant sometimes. When I heard this, I thought, 'That's my girl! Don't go down without a fight.' The other night I couldn't stand by and hear her remonstrating while they whisked her into her bathroom. I left and wandered about the corridor. It wasn't long until she was ready and although Zilla, her key worker, said, 'Irene, Rach's waiting outside,' Irene lay on her bed curled up, looking distant. It was as though the essence of who she was had been trespassed on. In her own way she was saying, 'Look what you've done to me.'

How did I react? The real reason I dread these review meetings is because I don't want to break down and cry in front of all those people. Somehow, I hold it all in, stiff upper lip, while they tell me that the love of my life cannot understand that what she has in her hand is her own faeces and not something to eat.

The other night I dreamed that Irene was at home, in our kitchen. She was on a visit and my usual little waking fantasy about her being looked after at home was floating around. But Irene herself told me that she needed to go back to the home; that it was nice being back in our house, but the best place for her was where she is now. It felt strong coming from her; she knew what she needed at this stage of her life – at least, in the dream she did.

There were three doctors at this review, a nurse, the occupational therapist, our CPN and a student nurse. Afterwards the OT gave me a sheet with some sort of assessment of Irene. She asked me if I thought it was accurate but the only word I could take in was, 'Irene'. All the rest was OT-speak and gobbledygook to me.

Our social worker had sent her apologies. I later found she'd been off sick. This was a real shame as the main information we need right now, about financing Irene's care and what the options are, is from her. Irene is also to be referred to someone for a nursing assessment, which I'm told if it's a level 5 will mean that her care will be paid for by the health service. Irene will also be referred to the continuing care co-ordinator. I now understand that the place where I left the penny won't be right for her. She needs somewhere which is more purpose built, with wide corridors, flat and more geared to her level of nursing need. So I need to start again, to find the right place. This feels like a massive responsibility, but for now, today feels like a milestone, a day to have got through.

Later the OT rang me to say that she had assessed Irene and she (Irene) had done well, whatever that means. She (the OT) was sweet and well meaning – and very young. She said it 'only' took two people to get Irene dressed. Oh no! I thought – we needed Irene to be worse than that as we need that level 5 assessment to get free care!

Well, can't do any more, out of my hands now. Just have to wait (again!) and see.

Christmas in the Half-way House

22 December 2007 Zilla said, 'I don't mean to be patronising but…isn't it awful – she's so young. Well, it's awful for you too, but she would have had so much life still to live.'

The elderly singer they had brought in for entertainment cracked me up with his first song, the lyrics something like 'I'll forget many things in my life but I won't forget you'. Maybe he thought this was the most appropriate song for an audience of dementia patients but I found it almost too painful. He carried on for about an hour with old songs and he went down well. Irene chattered mostly but made the staff laugh at one point when the singer threw his arms around theatrically and seemed to be pointing to a corner of the ceiling. Irene also pointed to the spot and said, 'Yes, it's up there'. She does make them laugh. Gordon was also tearful in places, and sentimental as he is, enjoyed the old songs. It was all pretty moving.

When I was leaving, I went to Irene's room to get my coat. Nora, a new patient said to me, 'Did you find what you were looking for?' I said, 'Yes,' though I hadn't been looking for anything, and she said, 'Will you help me to find what I'm looking for?'

23 December 2007 I was feeding Irene her second bowl of ice cream at the table in the corridor and Barbara, a patient, came and sat down near us. She's the one who always wears her coat and there's hell to pay if she can't find it. She started taunting, 'Why are you feeding her, she's nothing, she doesn't deserve you, you're a slave to her. She's nothing, she's from the back streets, she's a slut, a tart…' and on and on. I know she's ill but I thought, 'Any more and I will brain you'. I wanted to say, 'She's worth forty of you, you old cow and if you carry on I will kill you.' I managed to hold on, finish feeding Irene, then we got up and walked away. I didn't say anything to her but she really upset me. Irene didn't know anything of course, and she is so sweet and trusting. It seemed so unfair. If anyone hurt a hair of Irene's head I would give them what for. My God.

A shame, as we'd had a lovely day, a friend's tea party for Irene. I brought glasses and a bottle of sherry, mince pies, and we took over the blue lounge. Lots of our friends came and Irene was fine. She was very affectionate and responded to the fact that it was a social event. She understood, and she recognised some people. She sometimes needed to wander off, but she also sat with us for a long time and entertained people; at times she just looked like she used to, rolling her eyes, making faces, waving at people across the room.

When I arrived, she was really pleased to see me and said, 'Oh, oh Rach! Can we get married?' It upsets me to think that she might be upset about us not being together – she is aware of it, and asks me where I've been. She seems conscious of the fact we're not together. Otherwise why would she say things like, 'Why can't we be together?' or 'All I want is to be with you'. It hurts if she's distressed but on the other hand I like to hear her say that she remembers me and wants to be with me. I know one day remembering won't be there at all and I'm grateful to have it back after the haze she was in, in the Bedlam place. Sometimes, when I think of her dying, I feel a rising panic, a hard tight feeling in my chest, and I'm ready for the sobs to come. It's one thing to have her there, ten miles away where I know there's a spark of love between us; she's there. But the thought that she won't be there is unthinkable, a terror.

It's 4 o'clock in the morning and I can't sleep. I've set my laptop up in the bedroom – simple idea – don't know why I didn't think of it before. I have got stuck into habits but now I have the house to myself I can organise it how I want to. Not sure why I can't sleep, though I think of things, am aware of my mind working overtime. I'm very tired but I lie awake, or I sleep for a bit then wake again, and less than an hour has passed. I might not see Irene today – Christmas Eve now. I need to have a day when I don't go anywhere or do anything. I'm so tired.

The winner of *Strictly Come Dancing* was on the front page of the *Observer*. HAS the world gone mad?

25 December Happy Christmas sweetheart. It's 3.45 in the morning and I was wide awake and my brain working so I needed to do something and then maybe I'll sleep again. I spent Christmas Eve sorting out your study. I have cleared out a lot of books, mainly your more academic books on literary criticism, stuff I will never read. I also got rid of various poetry books, the more obscure ones. I have kept lots! And anything personal I have kept, like a French dictionary you were given as a prize at school, and a book with an inscription from your dad. Quite a lot were your old English teacher's, which meant a lot to you but nothing to me. I have made space and tidied up. I came across a number of your handwritten and private diaries and journals. It feels an invasion of your privacy to read them but I will read them, sometime in the future when it's less painful to do so. Some will be joyous, like your account of your cross-Sahara journey, but I know others are from your troubled times like when you had to give up teaching, and they are, from my brief glimpses, full of your angst. I came across an envelope of all the cards I've given you, for birthdays and anniversaries. That was sweet, though I couldn't look at them for too long. When I really cried was taking a card off the wall which I had painted, a Scottish castle which said inside that I would love you this century and the next, which was true. It must have been from that Christmas we spent at J's bungalow in Scotland, just the two of us, when we left the potatoes in the car overnight and they went frost bitten so we had a small ration of roast potatoes on Christmas Day. That year it was seven degrees below when we left Gordon's to drive further north.

This is the first Christmas you've not been aware of being with me in 28 Christmases. Feels strange waking up in bed on Christmas morning entirely on my own. I think this is the first time in my whole life that's happened. Goodness, I can see why Christmas is hard for people.

I wonder if you understand that it's Christmas. It's so hard not knowing what you know. I wonder if you ever consider where you are or why you're not at home. I wonder if you ever remember our home. I have no idea what's in your head, and that is strange after years of just knowing what's in your mind, (and you knowing what's in mine) without having to say anything.

I worked all day at clearing up but often I just have to stop and I stare vacantly into space, mesmerised with tiredness. I want to howl to the world the pain of not being with you. I'm here in our bed, knowing everyone is wondering if I'm OK, and you're a few miles down the road surrounded by kind strangers. I wonder if you're wandering the corridors or if you're safely asleep.

I will shed some tears and then I will read Dylan Thomas's *A Child's Christmas in Wales*; I found a lovely little version of it yesterday in your room. It's just that poem, with woodcut illustrations, costing 60p and printed in 1979.

Happy Christmas my love. I will see you later.

26 December   Am in bed, feeling a bit rough, a cold. I'd like to stay here. Can't quite believe Christmas Day is past, as it seemed such a milestone to get through. Irene was pleased to see me; she grabbed my hand and said, 'Oh come on, love, come on!' as if she wants us to go off together. She sat all the way through lunch without wanting to get up once. And we also shared some tears – usually it's just me – but she said, 'Why do you need to leave me here; can't we be together; I love you,' and more that I can't remember. And we just hugged each other and she was crying, her face contorted and wavering, and I thought I would cry forever but we didn't as she went back into her new self, and laughed and started to talk in the way she does now, her plinkety plonk talk, and then we both laughed and I talked plinkety plonk too.

She understood to pull the cracker and wore her hat for a while. Another patient, Joan, and Joan's husband were also at our table, in the corridor. He was losing it, couldn't get it at all, started to tell Joan off, not to be naughty, now sit down and eat your lunch, you've got to eat. And she was getting up and being vague and unable to respond. A helper came by and asked if he needed help and I mouthed, 'Yes!' and they came and took her into the dining room. He sat there tight-lipped and methodically ate his Christmas lunch. Later he was wandering around with Joan and then left, but before that, he said as he passed me, 'She told me to go!' and I thought, 'Yes, I'm not surprised, mate, people with dementia know what they want!'

I enjoyed feeding Irene and it was a good visit. Irene was telling me she wanted us to go off together. I hadn't expected so much of this, of her really understanding that we are not together. She sometimes asks me where I go. But then she also so easily goes off into her own new world. I do still have ideas about her coming home, of her being here, though I know that's a fantasy and neither of us would manage.

Dorothy, the new patient, kept asking me where the office was and how she could talk to the manager. I showed her a few times then really told myself it wasn't my problem. She kept asking me how she could go home. I told her I was just a visitor and she told me I was a liar. I wish I had Alan Bennett with me as he could turn all this into the most amazing play just by writing down the dialogue verbatim, and then we could co-produce it and I could get lots of money and not have to worry about paying for Irene's care.

Then I left – I'd been there nearly three hours – and went to my sister Penny's. I joked that I'd arrived at the madhouse and Penny's grimace told me that it was a madhouse. Christmas family horror show. By the end of the day Irene's place seemed the more normal. Penny had warned me that X's parents are truly awful and given her inability to cope with anyone for long I had expected some exaggeration, but they are – truly awful. Poor Penny took refuge in the kitchen and at 7 p.m. said only two hours to go – they had a taxi booked at 9. I escaped at 7 and went to bed as soon as I got home. Colds are sent to save us from ourselves sometimes.

The times at Irene's place are more real and more special than times anywhere else. It is indescribably painful when Irene tells me how much she loves me and I know she is struggling to understand why we are apart. This is more painful than the times she walks past me in the corridor and doesn't recognise me, bumps into me and says, 'Oh, sorry!' and walks on.

People have invited me to all sorts of things and my social calendar is full, but I need to stay in my wilderness until all the tears are out, I don't want to be rescued.

27 December   Sitting in bed at three o'clock in the afternoon with a cup of tea, and the music from *Brideshead Revisited* has just been on Classic FM. So resonant of that time in our lives; we used to watch it every week and play the music – an LP! Just had my daily blub. When will I feel any better? Ever? I want time to have sped on. Not seeing you today – sorry. Feel full of cold. I took a load of books to the Oxfam shop this morning and was going to see you after that but decided to put myself first which is what everyone tells me to do. It's more putting my cold first as I really want to see you but feel too lousy and don't want you to get it now I'm coughing.

Good visit to you yesterday, lots of cuddles and you knowing me, for an hour and a half. Also talked to a senior nurse who disclosed that Barbara is sectioned – Ha! I thought. He also gave some advice on how to handle it if she gives me grief again. She seems the sort who would be locked up for sending hate mail (or dog shit through the letter box) to her neighbours.

I feel bad not seeing you – am I hard on myself? I have set myself up to say, 'I go every day'.

What seems most left for you is your emotional memory – you know you have me and you know you have a special brother, though at times it seems anyone else can stand in for us, as you clasp strangers' hands too. You must have been a happy little girl, because that is what you seem to be now. Am hoping that if I write this now, it will all be off my mind and I can sleep. Have had paracetamol, whisky and am tired but it all doesn't help that much …

29 December   Am in bed. Whenever I feel poorly I can't decide whether it's a deeply symbolic visit from a guardian angel that means I can stop, lie in bed, feel sorry for myself etc. or whether it's just bad luck, I just came into contact with a bug and it got me this time…Well, whatever, it's a pisser. I do feel rotten and it means I won't see Irene today. The sun is streaming in so much that I can't see the laptop screen and all the dust in the house is shown in amazing detail. It's a dazzling day though also windy with occasional little squalls of rain. Takes rain and sun to make a rainbow so they say, a trite way to explain that we need sadness in our lives? Just reading Alice Walker's book *Now Is the Time to Open Your Heart*, quite a lot of New Age bull though it's OK for me to say that as a person of non-colour – a lot of it is about indigenous and black people recovering from the injustices of European treatment but it occasionally also contains some wisdom that seems to speak to me. And I wonder again, like I do about illness, whether the books we choose to read actually choose us. It's about a woman on a spiritual quest. Am I just in bed with a bad cold or was this sent to me so I can plumb the depths and really stop, literally stopped in my tracks so I can reflect and absorb what's happened to me? Could do without this ruddy cough anyway. And I'm pissed off I can't see Irene. I enjoy curling up with her. Yesterday I did just that, lying on her chest, hugging each other like old times, that closeness and warmth. Something we had temporarily lost and occasionally now have back. We can still do that. Oh, but it is a shadow of our former selves, a poor compensation really, but something at least. And I miss it if I'm not able to go there.

You were so pleased to see me, grasping me tightly, Paul and Colleen having just changed you in your bathroom.

I feel like I am being taken towards a door and, if I go through, will mean that my life on the other side will be forever changed. There will be no way back and I have to decide whether I want to go there or not. My face in the reflection of the laptop looked lined and grimaced. I am older, careworn, tired and looking my age. I have started to do things my mother used to do when she was living on her own and had no one else to check her behaviour, like swigging straight out of the cough medicine bottle or cutting toe nails and not bothering where the bits go, hearing them ping off the furniture. Oh dear. ANYWAY, THE OTHER SIDE OF THE DOOR IS LIFE WITHOUT YOU, WHEN YOU ARE REALLY GONE AND I WILL BE ON MY OWN, WITH YOU AS MEMORIES, PHOTOS, LAUGHTER, A PRESENCE BUT THE REAL YOU, IN YOUR BODY, GONE. Caps lock came on by mistake but maybe I'll leave it on – one of those things that either happened for symbolism or because my fingers are just too fat and clumsy ...

Is this what 2008 will be about, getting to that door? Or should I not even be thinking about that, but just enjoying what's left with Irene? Like they say when you have cancer, hope for the best and prepare for the worst?

I did feel better having gone out to the opera, that hopeful side of me that gets released when I don't spend too much time on my own, which is when I get maudlin and feel sorry for myself. I have sorted out quite a lot of stuff, made a trip to the Oxfam shop and one to the Help the Aged. And the dustbin men have been, taking away three great sacksful of stuff. The house is beginning to look less cluttered and I sorted through that great pile of letters and papers that were lying on the dining room floor. Found the new bank card which I've just had replaced as I was sure it had gone permanently to ground … I put it on the fire and was interested to see what happening to it, curling up and melting. I have taken stuff that once I was keeping as it seemed significant, like the vase we bought once from a local agricultural show – not sure I liked it that much even when we first bought it all those years ago. The surfaces are beginning to look clearer.

I guess some of this is about making the house mine, not just de-cluttering. I had not thought about needing to sort out Irene's things, which is obvious when you consider. Her personal things, her history. No use to her but not quite sure they belong to me …

Christ, I'm going to turn this frigging laptop off, stop being so bloody precious and just enjoy an afternoon in bed. Why am I so serious, sanctimonious? Am I the only person in the world with shit going on? Christ's sake, lighten up.

Lists

December 2007

1. **Things I have lost**

Our shared memories. Funnily enough, you were the one to remember things more and remind me of them.

Our future together, growing old together, seeing how you might be when you're 88 or 99. Our active retirement, our plans.

You to talk to, discuss things, make decisions. My sounding board, keeping me sane and on the level.

Your presence in our house.

Our relationship as it was; my soul mate. I still don't understand how this has happened. I can still be surprised that I found my perfect partner and you were taken away. Who wrote that script? Didn't they understand that what we had was so special, so rare that it was meant to have a happy ending? Is this how a twin feels when they lose the other? I have felt like half of a whole for so long that I feel now like what – a half? As if there is always something missing. Well, there is something missing.

Our way of life, all the things we would do together, walking, travelling, seeing friends. Funny how all I wanted in life was you – all the rest I would have happily dispensed with if it meant keeping you; job, money, house. We could manage anything if we had each other.

Being with someone I know so well and who knows me – so we don't have to talk, we just know. How to start that all over again with someone else? A quarter of a century of spending so much time with one person so that you can communicate without realizing it. Such hard work to get there and then it's all gone.

Someone to cuddle up to in the night.

Someone to make cups of tea on weekend mornings so I didn't need to get out of bed.

Someone who always had a spare hanky and would always give up her own to me.

A Happy Ending.

Oh, but could I have gone on in the way we were those last months? No. Your increasingly erratic behaviour, the tension of not knowing what eruption would happen next. That surge of relief once I'd got used to you being in hospital, the sheer joy of having survived, the realisation that I could cope on my own, I could climb Beamsley Beacon and savour the wonderful sunshine and be happy. But, oh – to go back six or seven years and have you as you were, that warm, loving funny personality who was mine, all mine, who I wanted to love till kingdom come. And I am crying now like there's no tomorrow because tomorrow is gone.

2.   Things I still have

The anticipation of seeing you. Your smile when you see me.

Someone who says, 'I love you' each time I see them. Our home.

My job.

Our friends.

My sisters and brother; your brother and sister-in-law.

My optimism and sense of joy and wonder in the world.

3.   Things I have learnt to do

How to keep warm in bed: You were always such a hot water bottle. You radiated heat. When you got up to make us both a cup of tea at the weekend, a job you did almost to the end, I used to move over to your side of the bed because it was so warm, whereas if I get out in the night for anything, my place is stone cold as if no one had ever been there. I would snuggle up to your back in the night, sometimes just for warmth but also to be next to you, a warm human body. I did change to one of our other duvets after you'd gone but two nights ago I started to use the one off the spare bed. (Regular guests will notice.) It must be the one we bought when we had the cottage at Garsdale, as it's that really thick one that I remember burrowing under up there, especially that cold, snowy winter of 1986. Remember sometimes we followed the snow plough, and we tobogganed down our road from

Cowgill, that steep bit. Anyway, we never did quite get the heating sorted and that duvet was lovely. I think it's synthetic but, whatever, it's doing the trick now and I am sleeping a bit better.

I found it strange that only two nights after you'd gone I moved to the middle of the bed. Strange as even in hotel rooms on my own I would always stick to my side of the bed, the left side that I had always been on. It seemed natural to move to the middle of our bed, as if I knew you were not coming back. I miss you.

How to make decisions:

Big ones: don't make them.

Small ones: decide what feels best and do one thing at a time. E.g. do I go for a walk as it's a nice day and then go to the supermarket and then go to the gym? Do I go to Sainsbury's where I could go to the gym afterwards (or am I too tired?) or do I go to Waitrose on my way to see Irene, so saving a journey (and carbon miles etc.) but what if I get stuff that needs to go into the freezer and I'm with Irene for ages? If I don't go to the supermarket how will I get A's present and can I face the supermarket anyway on the Sunday before Christmas? So many decisions and these are the ones I agonise about. So – what to do? Just do one at a time, i.e. go for a walk. By the time I get back time has marched on and I decide to call in at the farm shop, and really who needs food over Christmas anyway?

How to carry on alone:

Just got on with it.

4. Things I now understand

Why divorce is so painful: the loss of status, of a partnership, of learning to be on your own yet your partner is down the road or still around somewhere. Dealing with people as a singleton.

Why being able to say 'my daughter' or 'my son' is so special: Someone to call your own. And I put all my eggs in one basket, my all into Irene and me. I understand how decisions you make thirty years ago affect you now – well, I didn't mind all that but I feel wounded now when I see people all around with, it seems, everything; the family, the partner, the second home in the Dales, and they find it so easy to say, 'My daughter is home for Christmas' or 'When I visited my son' and they take it all for granted. And I feel I just have me – everyone else in my life has another person who is closer to them, who has more call on their affections than do I. Irene was mine and I was hers. That's what a partnership is and it feels like I gambled all my chips on one and in the end lost everything. It seems strange to describe it like that, like an investment which went wrong and I feel bad thinking about Irene like that, in such mercenary terms. And I know I still have all those things I did with Irene – I would never have been able to have such a life with anyone else, someone so in tune. How amazing it was to have found someone where we were so in tune, growing together over the years. I can't quite believe how in tune we were.

5. The Horrors

I need to write about the horrors, the things I can hardly bear to think about.

Being told about the diagnosis. Jesus, that was crass. Shock, bewilderment but also recognition of the unknown horror which had been growing in my mind. Now confirmed.

Sitting in our garden at the round table, and you pleading don't give up on me, will you, help me, help me. Knowing that you were going from me and you not knowing, not knowing it would only get worse, a descent into hell, and it was so awful, so awful and now all I can do is sob because it was about the worst thing of our whole life.

Driving to Scotland and you grabbing my arm and squeezing it so much it hurt and I was doing 70mph in the outside lane of the motorway and you were furious and like a demon. And then you were scared and stopped doing it because I was weaving over the road, not able to keep the car in a straight line and suddenly cars were giving us a wide berth. I managed to slow and pull over to the slower lanes though I didn't stop but kept on, having shouted at you and you realised it was serious and were quiet.

Me leaving you at Gordon and Pauline's house though they were out, because I couldn't stand it anymore and you were shouting at me to get out of the house. You didn't recognise me so I thought, OK I'll go. So I went and I knew where I'd go – to the pool in the next town, and I swam and swam. Afterwards I still wasn't ready to face you so I sat in the car and watched some young guys doing rugby training, passing the ball up and down the field, up and down. Then I drove but I still wasn't ready to face you so I stopped the car and sat where I had once thought I'd seen a short eared owl on the back road between Kippen and Callander, but I didn't see it. Then I did get home and I knew Gordon and Pauline would be worried so I drove up but couldn't get out of the car. Pauline came out and we talked. Later, you still didn't recognise me and when one evening eating dinner you asked where I lived and Pauline said, 'Why Rach lives with you,' you shouted and ran crying from the room and said, 'But she can't – I hate her, I hate her,' and on and on. You looked at me as though I was two people. You looking at your life partner as though she was perfect stranger, a dark person that you were scared of. How could that be? After a quarter of a century together? The shock dawning on me that you didn't know who I was.

Those last days at home, living a crisis and knowing it couldn't go on. Holding my breath, holding at bay the panic that it might not get any better.

Driving you to the acute psychiatric hospital, though I have written about that elsewhere. And I'm not going there again.

Thinking about you dying. It's one thing to know you're down the road, even if demented, and quite another to think that you might not be here at all one day. And how will it happen? Like in the movies, in my arms, all the important people around your bed? Or some other way? Why did this have to happen? Why am I on my own? Why couldn't we have gone on forever, enjoying our little lives, being content with coffees out and walks in the Dales?

Becoming my mother. Oh God – I do look more and more like her and Penny often said, 'Ooh, you looked just like mum then,' and I know I did, because I feel like her. I could not bear to end up like her, sitting on her end of the sofa for as many years on her own as she was with dad, living alone and with no one to be special to her. Apart from us that is, her children, but we sometimes went under sufferance and we had our own lives, though she was so proud of us – we became her life. I do not want to end up alone, lonely, going slightly batty. I want to love someone else, find happiness in mid-life and bumble around happily with another love. Is that someone out there? I guess they are as long as I can find them. But the thought of loving someone without Irene's face feels utterly alien and I wonder if I could. I'm scared that people feel sorry for me, that they don't ring because they want to but because they ought to see how I am. Or they don't ring at all and then I'm left feeling alone and that they don't care. Or they do ring and then I feel a bit pressured, that my silence where I can be with Irene in my head, and with my own unhappiness and sadness, is punctured. I always thought mum did well on her own, that really she preferred it, but maybe she was just making the best of a bad job – the only job available – just like I might have to.

A New Year

I have been doing more sorting out in Irene's room, in her study. I found lots of things which could make me cry but when I did really cry was when I came across a blue envelope with 'jewellery' written on it in her handwriting and there was a lovely little necklace and matching earrings which I vaguely remember her not being able to find at some point. I seem to remember her being upset that she couldn't find them and I'm pretty sure they were meant for me, so I'm wearing them now.

Lots of cards from me to her – lots of Valentine cards and all sorts of other things which I don't have the heart to look at now. So lots of stuff I just piled in her desk drawers. I seem to remember her starting to clear stuff out which is why the top of her desk was such a mess. Her room is getting clearer now to the point where I can think about moving in myself.

Am also finding it a bit difficult being with Irene – maybe I've just gone there too much or am tired or need some other emotional outlets in my life…Irene is a bit vacant at the moment, not as agitated and is more able to sit through a whole meal and also today I left her watching TV. I'm not sure she notices when I pop out. Gosh, this is so hard. I went to Penny's and literally had a cry on her shoulder.

Clearing Irene's desk I came across a book of Douglas Dunne's poetry, written after his wife died. It fell open at the poem 'Land Love' and my eyes went to the lines:

With all the feelings of a widower
Who does not live there now, I dream my place
I go by the soft paths, alone with her.

How perfectly apt. I feel alone with Irene.

3 January 2008   I'm sitting in your study looking out of the window, my laptop on the cleared table, and with that lovely view over the garden and then over the fields. The first time in 20 years that I've had this view to myself. You sat there all those years, wrote letters here, wrote your novel here, and all those sad journals too. The chair isn't quite the right height so I will need to see to that, but otherwise it's great. All your things are still on the corkboard, your photos and things you'd stuck up.

It's snowing outside and although I've been out I'm glad I'm back inside in the warm. I'm not visiting you as the ward is closed due to another outbreak of sickness...I felt better for a few hours yesterday, buoyed up by a successful shopping expedition to get you some new nightwear, as you seem to be managing to destroy your pyjamas. You tear them up somehow.

It's fantastic looking out on this new window on the world, watching the snow cover the green grass. Lots of birds around, I guess hungry.

I watched the Julie Christie film *Away From Her*, where she plays a Canadian woman affected by Alzheimer's in her early sixties. I'd expected a wracking experience but in fact it left me cold, except in places where the husband was stopped in his tracks, and I thought – I know how that feels. His pain was more real than her portrayal; or rather it was the story line that was so unbelievable – she decides herself to be admitted though to me she doesn't seem that bad. Then the husband isn't allowed to visit for a month (which no institution would recommend) and in that time she forgets him completely and gets attached to another male patient. The husband seems to team up with that patient's wife in a new relationship as the film goes on, and the whole thing is really a love story – about their 44-year marriage, about his past infidelities and their current devotion; about the wife in the second couple deciding to choose happiness over slavish devotion, and so on. The Alzheimer's was not life-like – even though it varies so much between people – and the nursing home was lively, everyone able to play cards, for example, and to move around quickly. It was a sanitised version of dementia and as such held no terrors for me. Julie Christie's dementia seems a fairytale cosy vagueness and not the dreadful, life-halting, crippling of personhood that it really is. It had little effect on me, whereas I'd expected a good cathartic clear out. I guess some of the husband's grief and alarm did ring true and did bring a few tears for me but then it seemed only a short while and there he is shacked up in bed with the other woman! Still grief-stricken of course, but life doesn't seem like that to me.

Anyway, I saw it in HMV and bought it. I didn't even think Julie Christie was that great in it, whereas people are saying she deserves an Oscar. I spent rather a lot in HMV, as is my wont these days. I bought the Frank Sinatra CD that was played at our civil partnership – the very same double album. 'Let's Face the Music and Dance' as we walked up the aisle, and 'The Best is Yet to Come' as we walked out. Well, brave to the end. The brave might not live the longest – but the cautious don't live at all, and we did some brave things together.

My – our – good old friend Tom was meant to be coming over but it's forecast snow all over England, the ward is closed due to this outbreak, and also they have found an unexploded bomb which means the M62 will be closed. All in all the runes seem to be telling us to change plans today.

I still have my cold and still feel like crap. On a day like this Irene would have gone out and larked about in the snow and maybe even have dusted off the sledge.

Will I always miss you? When will the pain of this stop? Early days, early days. I know it will take a long time but sometimes I wish I could fast forward my life and get through this and on to the things which will make me feel better. Have to stop now, as I'm too sad.

4 January 2008 Joan [someone I met at the Alzheimer's support group] has just rung to say that her husband Trevor has been admitted to the acute psychiatric hospital. Whew. I know how that feels. She is so sweet and kind, always asking me how Irene is, even though she must be in real pain just now. Anyway it came to a head with Trevor, who had got violent. Joan says he keeps asking to come home and a few nights ago a whole group of them all decided on a mass break out, so it took a long while to get them all settled again…She says how much she hates leaving him there when it comes time to go. All that with Irene feels like another life, and certainly was a different chapter. She really wants to keep in touch. She has a way of saying things which hit the nail on the head, and are said so simply, like, of our loved ones, 'Well, they're our life, aren't they?' when someone questions us why we are visiting them every day.

5 January 2008   Irene was sweet today, very happy, singing a lot. The occupational therapist Kathy said how lovely she had been, even when she was feeling unwell she was still singing. Today Irene said 'I love you so much, I don't know what to do with it all'. It bucked me up, the whole visit, as we sat and she was very affectionate and loving. We sat on the sofa in the corridor as her door was locked after they had cleaned the carpet…I like the special times when it's just Irene and me in her room on our own too, but somehow having affirmation from others, to be in public, makes me feel like we still have our partnership intact. She seems to be feeding herself more and also going into the lounges and sitting down. The staff all like her.

Her conversation goes something like this:

'Gordon, Gordon, come on, come on, let's walk, do do do do, dooo…' Then if I manage to sit down with her, 'Oh Rach, you are lovely, yes, lovely, and a pitcher pitcher pitch and yes well that's what I said said said ped ped pedipot, redipot, pot and we said yes let's go; shall we go for walk I'd like to go for walk with you, yes.' Then maybe a bit of a song. 'Yes, well, I said over there, that's right and a right right givey gone, givey gone and fed, fed, what's fed? On the ped on the fed on the sed and on the sed', then some more song. And then off again in the same vein. 'Yes, over there, isn't that lovely, and over there, yes I saw that, yes.'

It's one thing to get through what's happening, to go and see Irene, cope with it, all in the present. But it's the future that's hard, that I will always be without Irene, that the empty years stretch ahead and it will always be thus – that Irene is apart from me and I from her. It's hard accepting that this is it – forever without her. I guess this happens in any loss, you get through the shock and the knowledge of it but then it sinks in that this is really how it will be.

I found something Irene wrote before she became ill: '20 reasons to love Rach '. It made me cry, naturally. It was lovely too. She really did love me, still does, and that is what I really miss. Someone who really loves me, and only me. How wonderful that has been, to have in my life. I always knew that this would fortify me through the rest of my life, that I've had enough love to last a lifetime, but I still regret not having it for all of that life, still feel such a sense of loss that we no longer have our life together. It doesn't seem to be getting any easier. I feel a bit better now that I have the house in better order, have the rooms back so I can actually use them, but anything is small consolation.

6   January 2008   I don't know how to handle this grief in public. I know I chicken out when it comes to the crunch questions. I feel myself swallowing hard and backing off, changing to something less emotional, keeping it in. The other day when Cathy – nice Cathy from the village – met me as I was on my way for eggs from the farm, and she was saying how much I must miss having Irene around. Yes, you clod, I thought, and she persisted until I dissolved into tears. I don't necessarily want to be in tears in the lane going to buy eggs… but I also want people, to acknowledge what I'm going through. She only meant to be kind. I wonder how many times I've been insensitive, pursuing someone's obvious grief or unhappiness, in my clumsy attempts to empathise?

Got a big boost today as Tom [my good old friend Tom who Irene and I knew independently before we even met each other] drove over. Have not seen him since Irene and I went over to Cheshire – oh, how long ago? But old friends pick up immediately and it feels as though Tom's experience is most like my own – losing Robert, a special partnership, a long illness, a death and grieving. He really listened to me, explained that nothing feels right at the moment as nothing is right, everything is out of kilter because that's the way the world has become, and all my reactions to it are odd, suspect, and what is normal seems strange and my normality is what others would find unusual. Like a parallel universe, Tom said, and that is what it feels like, as others cannot see or really understand this parallel universe. So on Christmas Day it really did feel like I'd left a sane cosy place with Irene and gone to the madhouse at my sister's. Tom said it took him seven years to work through his grief, after Robert died. That's a long time and I wonder how long it will take me. I can see how you can have 'rebound' relationships, or attach yourself to anyone who shows some affection or attention. Dangerous but forgivable.

We also talked about not being able to get the right balance – seeing people or being on your own, for example, and always wanting the other, contrary to what you decided, and Tom said well there is no balance, it's all a struggle to keep in balance and being on an even keel isn't an option right now as the emotional seascape changes minute by minute. Difficult waters with no chart. Constantly making adjustments at the helm.

In the meantime I know I have to address finding a permanent home for Irene, and I will feel better once this has happened, the final piece in the care puzzle.

I have dismantled Irene's art room, our dining room, her pictures coming off the walls without even leaving grubby marks. I have put them all into folders, and will keep everything that she made during that last period of time at home. It's wonderful typing and looking out over the fields and the garden. It's OK to be on my own when I've had some good quality time with someone else. Tom talked about the mistake of cutting himself off from others, his life going in decreasing circles until he could face increasing those circles again. Maybe that's what I'm doing, plus protecting myself from people en masse or those who sap my energy.

7 January 2008   I have lost the love of my life, the thing I most lived for. Not surprising I feel so awful.

I now have a photo of Irene and me in every room, or one of just her. What a huge part of my life has gone. I still can't quite believe it. Why does it take so long to take this in? I can hardly believe I'm on my own. The times with Irene now in her new, temporary, home are still very special and I need them but I also know that my emotional mind is wandering and I need something else to fill this huge void.

I have chosen photos of Irene and me on the boat, as these were such special times, times when we felt alive, really alive. The photos look like we were really a team, doing stuff together. That was a happy time, and the times I really liked was just the two of us sitting on the boat, perhaps in the evening, especially when Irene was still well, and we would sit there outside in the cockpit, watching the stars come out. Or the days when we couldn't be bothered to sail, but would just sit in the sunshine and watch the world go by. I miss Irene as the person she was, the Irene of the photos before she became ill.

The house is somewhat reclaimed from the chaos, which means it feels more mine and more comfortable to live in, not the scene of a burglary or as if a hyperactive child has lived here. It was just a person with dementia and her carer, always too preoccupied to tidy up. I have got on top of the clutter, made numerous trips to charity shops with bags of stuff, dusted and collected a mountain of paper clips, plus put in one place all the postcards and other cards Irene bought over the years. I have enough never to buy any this decade. It all looks great though I haven't tidied Irene away – she's here in the corkboard on her study wall, all the bits and pieces she put up, and in the woolly bobble things she made, which hang in the kitchen and which, when I have time, I'll make into a mobile. And some of her paintings still hang in the kitchen. And the dreamcatchers she made with Chrissie. But I am alone, and alone I will be.

I weep and I need to weep until there are no more tears, but I can't imagine a time when there will be no more tears. So many tears, I can't believe how weepy I have been feeling. As if this deep well of grief is bottomless. I have no idea how deep it is, like looking into a black abyss. Deep dark water always did scare me, still does. I thought I would have got more used to the loss by now but it feels as though it's only just starting, not drawing to a close. And Irene is still there, a reminder of herself, the real essence of her still there.

Later – I have just been to see Irene and she was really on form tonight. I almost had a conversation. She was looking at the photos on her wardrobe door and said, 'That's a lovely photograph'. It was her dad she was talking about. She's often talked about her parents recently and also said she'd like to see my mother. I had a cry on the bed as she was hugging me tight. I can't stop the tears at the moment, probably why I couldn't face going into work today. Later as I watched her walk along the corridor, stooped over as she is now but still talking ten to the dozen, I could only wonder at where she has gone, compared with that person whose photo I have been plastering all over the house. The photo I have of us in 1985, where she is in the centre of the picture, no hint there of the person she is now. It suddenly hit me with a wallop just how she has morphed into another being, and although I can kid myself (and comfort myself) that her essence is there she is such a shadow of what she was, and of what she would still be if this had not happened. I cried all the way home, burst into floods as soon as I was out of there, and it continued till now. This is terrible, a terrible, terrible thing to have happened to someone who was so vital, so alive, becoming a stooped, mumbling and sad figure. Senseless, all senseless. She looks so great in all the photos, always laughing, always so alive. Why did this happen to such a wonderful person, so funny and alive and intelligent? She is at home there among the women who have been changed for the night, been walked back to their armchairs, or left to wander the rest of the day in the corridors before trying to get some calm in the place and get them to bed. The whiff of dirty nappies, the puzzled eyes – 'Can you help me?' And all the time Irene still seems so strong in her legs, could probably still walk for miles, and it was those legs which used to make me feel upset before she went away, as I knew I would really miss them, these long legs always ahead of me. Very thin now, and looking more like her dad when he got old.

And all the days without Irene stretching ahead of me and I wonder if I can do this, if I want to do this, go on without her. And I know I have to, I have no choice and from somewhere I will get a sense of purpose in life but right now I can hardly see the keyboard through the tears. I don't want grief to carry me away but I can hardly stand up against this flood.

10 January 2008   Am feeling a lot better today. The house has been full of people, almost each room filled with some activity and human warmth. Lovely to have the house used, full of chatter or just quiet bodies filling the space. And it's great that I have reclaimed it from chaos, so that I can enjoy looking at things, like the ash table we bought nearly twenty years ago from the workshop in Thirsk, and which has such lovely wood, which has been covered by Irene's paintings and art paraphernalia for many months. I wish I had taken a photo of it all before I cleared it up. I wanted to remember those paintings of herons on the walls, but I didn't want to keep the room like that. I don't want shrines to anyone though I have framed and put a picture of Irene in almost every room.

I had a great visit to Irene today. She was pleased to see me, and we sat and she ate a whole pack of melon and grapes and she chatted and laughed. It is so poignant when she makes a gesture just like she used to, like a flourish as she puts something in her mouth, just as she always has. It is so like her yet now she is so unlike her. It brings tears to my eyes to see it. She can be very funny, rolling her eyes, and pulling faces. I do the same, and we laugh. I have got used to being vigorous with her, tickling her or poking her in the ribs, and also talking nonsense, which she laughs at. After her usual hour, she needed to be off, walking the corridors again, forgetting me.

I was pleased, as the last visit was not good – Irene initially seemed to recognise me but then pushed me off, as if I was interrupting her, and she could not leave her world to come into mine. I left after a short time, as it does me no good, and her neither, probably. It almost makes it easier though, to get on with my life, when she's like that.

I realise it's a traumatic thing to see Irene in the ward, and also the other patients. A couple of times recently I have just watched Irene as she careers along the corridor, so bent and talking to herself, and the horror of it washes over me, threatening to topple me over, like a surprisingly small amount of water (knee deep) can. I feel traumatised by how quickly all this has happened, still only six months since we were in Holland, having a beer in the streets of Amsterdam, and later cycling along the side of the Rhine, and to see Irene now there is no comparison. This same person smiles at me from every room: her as May Queen at 17, in her old study, us in a photo booth fooling around, her on the High Route from Chamonix to Zermatt, and us sailing. There is no seed of any mental illness in those photos. Only in the one on our Italian disaster does she look vacant, as if caught unawares, not having much clue what was happening. Even in the Scottish disaster she can look perfectly normal. Then there are the photos I took recently, where she looks older, thinner and clearly ill. She looks better now, I think, than then, more relaxed. Oh dear, where have you gone, dear, dear one?

I am getting my act together a bit more again. I am no longer literally floored and can imagine actually doing some work, though again this morning I could hardly get myself out of bed. I have to talk to myself, tell myself come on, come on, get up. I could sleep for England. And I could cry for England too.

I also realise that if I knew for certain that I would meet a lovely woman in the future who would love me too it would make me feel a lot better. A lot of this is about Irene and losing her but I know it's also about losing someone, and if I had another someone at some point, I would feel tons better. Sometimes I think I won't ever love anyone who isn't Irene – and also who would love me?! – and other times I think I will definitely meet someone, and I have little scenarios in my head about how this might be, like the hopeless romantic I am. (I watched *Notting Hill* yet again the other night.) I do feel strange, like I've lost my twin, like I'm doing everything with my left hand and soon, at some point, I will go back to doing everything with my right hand again, and it will all feel normal. Except this won't ever be normal again because Irene won't be back. The other day I was sitting at the kitchen table, as I do, and I wrote on an envelope, 'I looked up and I hoped I'd see you walking into the kitchen like you used to'. But of course you won't. You are eight miles down the road yet a million miles away in your head. I'm not very good on my own, makes me go a little nutty. I so loved being a couple, the comfortableness of it, that slipping into step with each other without having to explain anything. And I would happily have spent 60 years with you, feel envious now if I hear of others who have been married for 60 years. I so wanted to grow old with you. I would have looked after you, and you me, both growing dotty and doddery together and, I'd hoped, dying together when we were very old indeed. We did have lots more life ahead of us – how many people have a good 20 years left when they are 60 – which seems so young nowadays? So many things we could still have done. And I feel I have lost the last five or so years too, as the dementia closed in and closed down our world. And it was so hard, organising everything, keeping you happy, and the emotional strain of it all, not being able to share it with you, losing you without being able to say things to you. Who do I say it to? The lump in my throat is threatening to close my throat so I cannot say it now, but that's what I need to do.

And tomorrow I have to go and look at nursing homes for you. I've been told we need an EMI one – elderly and mentally infirm. Never thought my life would come to this, looking for a nursing home for you when I'm 53. It's too hard. Cooking for one was the book we bought your dad after your mum died aged 77. He did so well for 11 months and then he died too. He was 81. He had 20 more years than you, still cycling to the end. Bastard fate.

Recently I've been aware that I'm conscious of my whole life, that I've thought about things in the past much more than I normally do, as if I'm aware of a whole chapter, rather than just living in the present. It's because the chapter is closing.

I still catch myself thinking that she will be here as normal – still!

It suddenly comes into my head that it's all different, 'Oh yes, I remember, you're not here'. Like a catch in my throat, a sudden memory. I find myself being unaware for a few seconds and am happy, and then I remember and I am instantly sad. I am so very alone without you.

14 January   Had three days of feeling OK again, that I'd not got a cold, and then bingo, Sunday evening I start to get a terrible sore throat. Tonight I'm meant to be seeing a film but I've not even gone to see Irene. I saw our GP and have some sleeping tablets. She said I was sensible and wouldn't get addicted. She didn't check that I might take them all at once, but maybe 20 wouldn't kill you. How I would love to do something that wasn't sensible.

Last night in bed, in the dark, I could have sworn that I could hear someone breathing out from time to time. Your presence is so real and we slept in the same bed for so long that I felt I could reach out and you would be there, and I would turn over and snuggle up to your warm back, snuggled up together against the world. I did actually put my arm out, just to check, but I knew you were not there.

I cannot sleep. You are on my mind all the time, whether you're OK, where you are going to live, whether you will be happy. It's not even a detailed thinking through of all this, more a general sense of uncertainty and anxiety that keeps me awake. I have done all the tricks – calming bath, candle lit, and sometimes a whisky, or a milky drink, and then reading till I can't keep my eyes open, and then bang, once the lights are out I'm awake. I lie in the dark and I want to cry, so I do, but that doesn't help either. A few great sobs, almost a panic of grief, and then I relax again but sleep doesn't come – until the dawn hours, soon after which I'm supposed to get up. Getting up is a great effort, and I have to really tell myself to move. Today it was 9 o'clock when I managed to get myself out of bed. I know I'm not well again, with this cold, but even so …

I will feel a lot better when all the arrangements are made – all very well for the social worker to say that costs can be negotiated, that there will probably be joint funding and so on, but I want to KNOW. I feel like my head is being squeezed, that I'm under pressure. Where will my love be? Will we be able to pay if need be and will I have any of Irene's income to go towards running the house? Will she be properly looked after? Will the place we decide on be right for her? Will we have much choice anyway? Will we be able to do all this before my work takes me overseas again? Will Irene remember me after I've been away for two weeks in March? That really scares me! Part of me wishes I was not going but a lot of me knows I must. I am ill now and I might get really ill if I'm not careful. There is a huge gap between what I want to do right now and what I've got the energy for.

17 January 2008   It's been raining for days, heavy rain about which there have been Met Office warnings. The ground is saturated and more rain is streaming down the road outside. It matches my mood, as if the earth could cry and cry. I feel better having found a place for Irene and I actually slept reasonably well, though helped with a little pill…

I still feel unwell and know I'm vulnerable to really going down with something. I have not got dressed, as though I need a badge to show I'm poorly.

23 January 2008   Every book I read has something which speaks to me in a deep way about my experience. This from Joyce Carol Oates, *The Falls*…

'…*to matter. To matter deeply, profoundly to someone. Not to be alone. To be spared the possibility of knowing oneself, in aloneness…Who I am there's no doubt. No longer. I know.*'

With dementia that certainty that you matter profoundly to someone is shaken. Irene has formed some type of attachment to someone else; the ward tells me there's been an incident, it happens sometimes. Actually it's that someone else – Margaret – thinks Irene is her husband, and though I joked, 'Good job I'm not the jealous kind', I did feel hurt, Irene's affection scattered anywhere, rather than at me.

24 January 2008   Am drinking a large gin and tonic. I needed a drink when I got back from seeing Irene. I sobbed in the car and had to wait for an interval before I could drive home. There was a huge full moon rising over the ridge and Beethoven's First Piano Concerto on the radio and it was so beautiful I almost stopped. But I carried on. What made me cry was Irene hugging me tight in the corridor and saying, 'Oh, Rach don't leave me. You are all I've got'. It really cut me up, and of course I did leave her, in the care of a nurse who needed to see to her nappy, which seemed to have slipped down her leg. And as soon as Irene had had this heart stopping moment of clear speech, she wandered off again in her mind, and laughed at something and was incomprehensible again, as if for her too it is too painful to dwell in the real world for too long, a glimpse of what has really happened, and then forget it again, quick, as this is too heart-breaking. She is so thin when I hold her. Now I want to cry as if there is no tomorrow.

I know I do matter profoundly to her and that spark keeps me going, but knowing that I matter so much yet I have to leave her there is killing me. If she completely forgot me, and I was no longer her special one, I would be distraught too. I am sitting here in her old study surrounded by her things, photos of her at about five years, sitting on a camp bed in a garden, her in her twenties in a small black-and-white photo, and her with Gordon, when she looks fine but we were beginning to think she was more than simply a fiftysomething with a menopausal memory, on the cliffs in Galloway.

They said today she will be assessed on Monday by the nursing home. As I was leaving, Irene had her hand on the nurse's shoulder, and then she was straightening the nurse's bra strap through her T-shirt, just like she used to do with me, one of those little intimate tasks, like picking a speck of fluff off someone's collar, that you do to your partner, and which tells you, if you see it in public, that they are probably married. I miss that easy intimacy, the unspoken communication, the ease with each other where you just fit in that comes from years of being beside that person. And I really value being able to say, 'We have been together 27 years,' or whatever. As if length really does matter. Lonely here on my own, lonely without you. I would give anything in a flash if I could have you back.

A Week's a Long Time in the Finding-a-Care-Home Game

January 2008

A week's a long time in politics but it's even longer in this game.

Friday   We had a follow-up meeting to the review, necessary because at the last minute our social worker couldn't make the CPA [Care Programme Approach]. So, our CPN, social worker, charge nurse, friend Jean and I met in a small room in the day ward. All very amicable, good round-up of the issues, not as daunting as the big CPA review on 20 December where there were three doctors, the OT, nurse, student nurse, CPN – and me. There is agreement that Irene is ready to be discharged to a new, permanent home. Good. There's delays in getting Irene's nursing determination done, which would be an assessment to see if she qualifies for health care (as well as social care), which of course would be good for me, and for social services. Nothing really has moved since the December meeting, as we need the nursing determination done and also a referral to continuing care and the financial assessment for me to go through Irene's finances.

After the meeting Jean and I head off to visit a nursing home which offers EMI care. I am sulky and don't want to like it as I can't bear to think of Irene ending her life in such a place. Anyway I make an effort but I don't feel comfortable – I don't tell them it's for my partner. It's run by a Methodist foundation and immediately my prejudices left over from childhood and my mother's church creep in and colour my views. I warm to it in the end more than Jean, who didn't like the chief nurse's attitudes.

We go home, as we need a cup of tea. I need a double brandy but resist.

Saturday   I was meant to go to another care home but they called to say they had the dreaded Norovirus so could I cancel. Instead I called on spec at another home near to where Irene currently is. They were welcoming and said I could have a quick tour. But I knew almost instantly that Irene wouldn't like it – fine if you are relatively confined and extremely sociable but I know Irene would be claustrophobic – not enough space for her to charge up and down.

Tuesday   I check when the nursing determination will be; Friday 1 pm, I'm told. Great. Feeling rotten with another virus myself. Not sleeping. Lots of things on my mind.

Wednesday   Planned to have been working at home but electricity cut off. So I decided to call the place I was meant to visit on Saturday; spoke to a nice man who said sure, come along. So drove – 10 minutes, that's all, which is promising. Nice man turned out to be Micky, who I suspect is gay. Anyway felt able straight away to say this was for my partner. He made me a cup of tea, talked to me, got to know what was needed. Had huge amount of confidence in the nurse in charge of where Irene will be who toured me round and told me how they try to amuse people and it all sounded really person-centred. Lots of bright décor, nice touches, very respectful of who people are and of what they have become. Rather alarming that everyone seems so much older than Irene, and some are very ill indeed, immobile on day beds, and one who likes to sleep on the floor. The main thing though is that there's lots of room for Irene to walk. She walks up and down all the time. I gather some people with dementia do this, and there were others doing the same here, walking up and down the corridors all day long. Anyway, came away feeling much happier. Got on the phone to social worker and said yep, this is it, can you phone them and get Irene assessed. Felt reassured about what she said regarding finance – that yes, they would fund this if health didn't do joint funding. I wouldn't have to find a shortfall or anything. Also talked to our CPN and updated her. She will chase up various reports after the nursing determination. Slept much better. Feel we have made two steps forward, finally.

Thursday   Didn't see Irene. Nursing my sore throat, and anyway she had four other visitors, one of them my sister, whom she told, 'Not today, thank you' – twice.

Friday Zilla stops me when I'm visiting Irene and says that they have started Irene on the Amisulpride again due to her aggressive behaviour – she has kicked people and slammed the bathroom door on them. They will not do the nursing determination today and also no nursing home will take Irene like this. I am stunned. I walk with Irene and we go to her room, where I shed tears, leaning on her shoulder. We have a happy hour and 40 minutes, with Irene being sweet with me though obviously telling angry stories, a lot of crossness about whatever she is feeling. Feel this is two steps back, to where we were a week ago. Am also upset that Irene is again on Amisulpride as I didn't think this did her much good last time, and also it seems to have happened without my knowing, and then I'm just told in passing in the corridor. Back home there's a message from the CPN, who has rung as she's also found out. She is frustrated and upset for me. The nursing home where I hope Irene will go was meant to assess her this morning but that has been cancelled too. They have vacancies and I just hope they can save her a bed.

I feel there's nothing else I can do and I need to relax again, go with the flow, accept there's not a lot I can do. Realise this is why the Serenity Prayer is in the ladies' loo in the CUE unit – accept the things you can't change. But I'm worried about Irene being put on a drug for what is really normal behaviour, i.e. to lash out if three people bear down on you, get you in a small space and start taking your clothes off. Especially if at that point you are eight years old and your mum and dad are still at work and you're home alone ... or whatever it is that Irene is thinking. She only behaves like this when certain staff are on duty, it seems to me.

I will just have to wait for next week, nothing I can do now. The CPN is going to that nursing home anyway on Monday and will talk to the lovely Karen who is in charge. Maybe we can put Irene's name on a bed while all the other mess is sorted out?

In the afternoon went to a consultation meeting organised by social services on reorganisation of mental health services for older people. Tried to get across the point about needing residential care for younger people with dementia ... but I think they just thought I had a personal beef.

Weekend Visit

By the time of my last visit to Irene in the community unit, she had been there three months. That shows how difficult it is to find appropriate care for younger people with dementia. My diary entry shows how hard it is to visit – to cope with other residents/patients as well as dealing with your own stuff. This home was built in a circle, the bedrooms off the corridor. So if you walked around the corridor you came back to where you started. It was less bleak than the acute psychiatric ward but still bleak enough.

Saturday 2 February 2008

Irene was crying when I arrived, wandering along the corridor. She was full of misery, tearful. I was shocked, as I haven't seen her like that. She kept stopping and whimpering with incoherent words. I called out to Colleen and she said that Irene had been tearful at lunchtime. I steered her towards the pink settee in the corridor near the nurses' office and by then I was in tears. I thought I'd lose it completely, as it was so heartbreaking to see Irene upset without knowing why and being able to do nothing. She said 'All I want is to be with you', and then, even more heartbreakingly, 'You're always on my mind'. She's never said that before, and I thought, oh, your poor mind.

And I was crying, like I'm crying now, and then Barbara came along, the one who is sectioned. She was agitated and insisted there was a problem across the road and can you call the police please? I directed her to the office but she came back again and insisted I help. I just wanted to be with Irene at this heartbreaking moment but knew Barbara wouldn't say no – it was all because Margaret kept going into Maggie's room and she and Barbara were getting aggressive wanting her out of there. So I reluctantly broke off from Irene and went to tell some staff, then back to Irene. I tried to cheer her up. She was very hungry and after two cookies, a piece of cake and two cups of coffee she was a bit happier.

Audrey kept wandering by, talking to herself and supplying her own answers. 'Well, what's in here. I don't know. Shall we try getting out up here. I don't know, I've no money and no food'. And so on, and Joan would also shuffle up, Irene eyeing her suspiciously as Joan fumbled along the chairs of the settee. And I was struggling with my love for Irene, feeding her calories and noticing how thin she's got. Eventually I needed more privacy and Irene needed to walk, so we went to her room, and I put another shirt on her as I thought she was cold. She has a cold and doesn't seem to be very well. She cheered up and then I noticed Irene's diaper down near her knee and two seconds later it emerged from the end of her trouser leg.

Another moment where you could laugh or cry. So I went in search of Colleen, who was sorting out someone's glasses. A new patient had someone else's glasses on and was laughing about the fact that she couldn't see. Fortunately they had the rightful owner's name on, Vivian, so they were returned and hey presto new ladies' glasses turned up too. It was funny and sad. So Colleen and another helper changed Irene, in a matter of minutes, and she emerged, wandering off again, having forgotten I was there. Then we met up again, and she was pleased to see me as ever. I was getting tired and caught myself thinking in a welter of guilt, England are kicking off against Wales at 4.30, first match of the Six Nations and will I be home? Or should I really stay with Irene, cheer her up some more? So we walked around the corridors again, and from the laundry there was wonderful fifties music playing, and I tried to dance a little with Irene but I'm not sure she really noticed. And some of the lyrics wrenched my heart. They seemed so pertinent, as so many songs are, about losing the one you love. So we sat again on another sofa and Irene chattered happily and put her arm around my shoulder and made herself laugh at her own words, and said whoops when she said shitty something, and we both laughed, as did the carer sitting nearby. They all can't help loving Irene, captivated by her personality and her obvious character.

Then I left as she was forgetting again that I was there. The road home was blocked by an accident, closed so it must have been bad, so I had to make quite a detour. And I thought, as I often do when I see an accident, what if I had been passing at that moment, instead of this one? So I got home, lit the fire and had only missed five minutes of the rugby.

Sunday visit

I decided to go early, for lunch time, so that if Irene was upset again she wouldn't have too long to wait before I saw her. She seemed OK, a bit less aware of me than yesterday, called me Gordon when I arrived, though later she used my name. She was fine, ate well, two puddings! As soon as she went into care, she seemed to lose understanding of using a knife and fork, and I feed her or else she dives in with her fingers. I don't understand this, as others seem capable of feeding themselves fine. She was quite communicative and kept putting her arm around me. My problem was another patient, Renee, who, as she was upsetting other patients in the dining room, was put opposite us with a carer to help her eat She is clearly suffering and the nurses were very concerned. She sounded awful and made me want to gag; reminded me of *Sweeney Todd* which I saw last night. Sorry but can't help thinking this. All the awful sounds the victims made when they had their throats cut; Renee made just that noise, but worse, kept bringing food back up. I couldn't look and just concentrated on helping Irene. Renee looks terrible. If Irene ever got anything in the night like food poisoning, she knew she was on her own! Yuck. I was always hopeless in that regard. Later I tried to clean Irene's teeth but she shouted loudly at me and I gave up. I felt chastised and she didn't seem too bothered that I was there by then so I left and went for a walk round the tarn. Seems ages since we both learned to sail there, the start of our sailing lives. Now there are interpretation boards every few hundred yards, in case anyone can't recognise a Canada goose. A few pochard among the more urban birds and a solitary Muscovy duck, looking alarmed. Felt better today about going away; easier when Irene is less affectionate, less aware.

Missing you

16 March 2008   I miss you in the morning, no one to take a cup of tea up to – and no one to bring me one. I miss you in the supermarket, no one to share it with and buy our stuff. I miss you all the time really. I miss walking with you. I miss snuggling up to your back in bed at night. I miss you in the car, driving along, and I miss talking to you. How long ago was it that we really could have conversations? All the things we did together, and now I can't plan anything with you. I miss you in the house, just being here. Feels so big and lonely now. There are photos of you all over it and you're not here. You never will be here again. Things will never go back to normal, things will always be out of kilter. I miss you saying you love me, miss having someone I can call my own, someone who is really mine and I am yours. Everyone around me seems to have someone and those who don't seem to want someone and are lonely, like me. How to manage on my own?

Miss you darlin'. Miss you, miss you, miss you to infinity; miss you with every part of me; miss you till I die. Miss you whenever I see the stars, especially Orion; miss you when I see all the places around us – all of them hold memories of you and me. Miss you being funny, your personality, your humour, your wit, your love, your touch, your hugs, your laugh, your awful singing. Miss you by my side, miss you like you're a part of me and I feel half of a whole. Miss our memories and our remembering. Miss having someone to share our past with; no one else knows what we knew. I have lost the memories. Miss having someone who always had a spare hanky and who would always share it. Miss my partner, my partner in life. Nothing can make up for that. I would trade anything to have you back as you were before this disease, maybe the you of eight years ago, or ten. I would give up the house, my job, all our money, I would go to live in Siberia if we could be together. But it won't happen and you will be there down the road and I will be here and I will see you every other day – I'm sorry darlin' but I can't manage every day. It is too hard and I feel too emotionally bruised by it. Why did you say 'It's me' in such a clear way? You were telling me you were there. To say 'It's me' – it's amazing. Where do you think you are? What do you think is happening? I cannot fathom it. I will never understand it, I will never be able to follow you. And when we could still cycle together, you used to wait for me on the top of the hill, and I would cry to myself, unknown to you, and I would think 'Will you still be waiting for me on the hill?' and I still wonder that, will you be waiting for me on the hill?

I will never desert you, I will look after you to the end, I will always be there. And you will be there as much as you can and you will look after me too because that is what you have always done and that's why you said, 'It's me,' because it is still you; you are there in some way and you look after me.

17 March 2008   Well, Irene did know who I was, even though I'd been away for two weeks, and keyed into me immediately. Karen said she knew I'd been away. We had three hours of good quality time. She said 'I love you' at one point and later, when we were sitting in the lounge and everyone else had gone to the dining room, she looked me in the eye and said with great precision, 'It's me'. I knew she was saying it was her, she's there – and part of her still is. It made me cry, and earlier too I was crying when we were sitting together in the garden room and she seemed happy. She also said a few things like she used to, like 'horrible' pronounced 'horrib–ley' – just as we both used to sometimes. It was uncanny.

And the house is full of her yet empty of her. Her. I see her more clearly now after a period away and I know I am alone here. I made myself go out to Chrissie's party which she had kindly invited me to. No longer part of a couple, I seem to find myself exploring new social worlds. This was one – I met such a different group of people, mainly artists who live in caravans and who make me feel incredibly bourgeois for having a snug, smug home. Her house is an eco house with a long drop loo and was built by a guy who lives in a sauna (he says) in the garden. Next door is a green architect. My feeble attempt to recycle and have a brick in my loo cistern, etc etc looks like tinkering with the deckchairs and my house seems like a palace. Chrissie has one room rented in a house shared with a young family. Jackie has just been on a spiritual pilgrimage to Peru where she had to eat bitter roots for six weeks and now she's back is uncertain how to make a living as she realises she has to give up her pottery work. Not a great deal of money to be made in being a spiritual healer here, I gather. My salary seems a fortune.

Anyway, good for me to get out of my groove and I realise I need to be more sociable, be with more people, be more occupied. If I can stay well then I can stay busy or at least occupied and, fortified with my contact with these creative people. I am going to make the branches I cut down from the bush near the pond into some kind of woven animal, bring out the creativity that must be lurking there.

24 May 2008   Yesterday as we walked outside in the grounds you stopped and said 'I hope you will be happy' and I was stunned and said 'Are you happy?' and you said, 'Yes.' How can you be so out of it, demented, and then suddenly say something which is so right, and how can you say things which tell me that you know we are special and yet we are apart? How can these two things, two states of being, co-exist?

I need to see you at the moment as I miss you so much. We hug a lot as you seem to be going through a patch of knowing me. You don't know I have an interview for promotion but what does that really matter anyway? I would give anything to have you back.

26 June 2008   I feel as though I have just limped off the battlefield after the war, not just the last battle. The war years of Irene at home becoming more and more demented. And I have lost.

I have lost Irene.

I feel I am sitting on a small rise looking down on the scene of the battles. I am weary and sad and wiser. I have been through all that, I have lost and I am alone.

I thought this stage would be where I moved on but I realise I am only just beginning to take in what has happened, all the traumas of daily life, the abrupt admission to the hospital, the rough leave-taking, the struggle to get the proper care – let alone beginning to recover. The scene up here is desolate. Every day I wake up and I think: 'Another day without Irene'. Another day without Irene. Another day without Irene. And I wonder if I can bear that, if I want that. Of course I don't but I will have to find a way to endure.

Being unwell is beginning to scare me. It would not be surprising to have colds one after the other but it would also not be surprising if I did get really ill with something and I fear that. I need to take action myself – bought monster vit C tablets yesterday. The weight I feel in my chest could be grief. This is like a weight that stops me breathing, a feeling that I'm holding my breath. And I do hold my breath. My upper chest is held tight all the time. That's where you feel the grief, there in your chest. And the rational in me says maybe it's hay fever. But I have had a succession of colds, things hit me hard. They say widows and widowers are more likely to die soon after their partner does. But Irene hasn't died; she's there but I've still lost her.

I do not want to be like Queen Victoria, (who certainly did live a long time after Albert) and I am not. But leading a double life, inward grieving, outward coping, has a price.

Another day without Irene. At least today I will see her. Make me feel like we are together, a whole, again. The battle separated us. I am dreading 29 August, the first anniversary. Feels like the day we were taken apart. When the real pain began.

Happy Days

11 July 2008   Irene loved to go to the theatre. We saw lots of big names – Maggie Smith and Margaret Tyzack in London in *Lettice and Lovage*, made all the more wonderful as we saw them strolling along the street to the theatre together, gossiping and obviously enjoying each other's company; Ian McKellen in a season at the West Yorkshire Playhouse, where he did three or four plays, all terrific; Kenneth Branagh in many Shakespeares in Stratford; Fiona Shaw in *Electra*, and our own (I mean we both had a crush on her) wonderful Helen Mirren in *Cleopatra* with Alan Rickman. We were so in love with her that we went down after work to London. We stayed at St Paul's youth hostel and caught the train back the next morning to get to work. And so many more. Prunella Scales in Beckett's *Happy Days* and she was amazing, especially as we caught the performance where she stayed afterwards for a discussion with the audience.

And *Happy Days* feels a bit like Irene's plight in reverse, a slowing down, a capture; her character keeping physical movement but losing her clearness of mind and Beckett's character losing all movement, progressively being covered with soil until at the end she's literally in it up to her neck, yet keeping a sharpness of the mind that is devastating in her blind stoicism. And there is a line which goes 'To have been always what I am and so changed from what I was'. And that applies to both Irene and me. We are both what we were yet we are also so not what we were, so utterly changed, me without her and she without her mind. Yet she is still her, the glimpses which are plain for anyone to see, the mannerisms, the way she laughs. And I am also so what I was, the me that has always been, yet my world is so different. I am alone and cannot get used to it.

I have those terrible compulsions when I'm driving and there's a juggernaut speeding towards me, and I want to swerve in front of it, accelerating. I know it's like the feelings you have at a sheer drop or waterfall, those feelings that it would be so easy to jump and you know you wouldn't if it came to it. But on the other hand the speeding lorry scares me as I know it's an easy way to relieve the pressure in my head, and that's what it's about. If the pressure ever got really great, I might just do it, and that is scary.

I read a poem by Brenda Lismer which helped me a bit:

There is an end to grief
Suddenly there are no more tears to cry
No hurt nor break now
But mute acceptance of what will be
Knowing that each move for good or ill
Must fit the whole
Past comprehension
Yet trusted in the design
This way lies peace.

I can't imagine having no more tears – I seem to have an ocean of them. It would be the Pacific Ocean. How many tears would that make?

I'm writing in what was Irene's study and her things are still up on the walls. There is a corkboard, made of actual corks cut lengthways so that they can stick flat on a board. There is a picture of her as a five-year-old sitting on a camp bed somewhere, her hair gripped to one side; a small black-and-white photo of her as a teenager, a lovely toothy grin and her fringe in her eyes; a picture of her nephews James and Daniel in school uniform aged about five and seven; a picture of her parents sitting in the shade on the ground, smiling; a strip of four photos of us in a booth in York station wearing large spectacles which cover half of our cheeks, dating it to the 80s. We are clowning about, both squeezed on to the stool and posing after we had done the proper passports shots. There's a lovely one of her and her brother, taken perhaps in 2005, posing on a cliff top in the Scottish borders, with no idea at all of the awful tantrums and upsets of the morning before they arrived. Irene had just been awful, shouting and arguing in a way that is not really about anything but is about everything, and I feel so bad now because I did not realise it was part of an illness pattern and that when everything became too much she would have no let out but to be bad. It was awful, her refusing to carry on walking; I cannot even remember what we said. All I remember is the awfulness, of being in the middle of a kind of madness. There's a picture of her which I snapped without her being aware; she is bent listening to her dad, he presumably telling one of his long anecdotes. We are on the Coniston steamer and it is after her mum died, when he so bravely carried on and learnt how to cook. There's also a special one of Gordon, posing against a wonderful Scottish backdrop on a long walk; her brother who was so special in Irene's life that she ran away from home aged eight when he was sent to boarding school as she was so disturbed by it. Now, she sometimes confuses me with him and calls me Gordon. And there is, on a piece of white paper, in her handwriting, 'Only love matters in the bits and piece of a person's life, William Trevor'. It's something she believed and something which she has left me.

The only other written piece is typed, attributed to Nelson Mandela:

Our deepest fear is not that we are inadequate. Our deepest fear is that we are powerful beyond measure. It is our light not our darkness which most frightens us. We ask ourselves who am I to be brilliant, gorgeous, talented and fabulous? Actually who are you not to be? Your playing small doesn't serve the world. There's nothing enlightened about shrinking so that other people won't feel insecure around you. We are all meant to shine as children do… And as we let our own light shine, we unconsciously give permission for other people to do the same. As we're liberated from our fear, our presence automatically liberates others.

There are lots of postcards, one of Andy Goldworthy's installations, a line of stones rising from water; two of a mother and baby zebra – she loved zebras, one of our most special days ever, when she saw her first, on the way to Cape Point below Cape Town; a photo I took of a big cloud of poppies, which she loved; several mountain scenes, including one of the Victorian walkers on the slopes of Mont Blanc, another of our favourite places, the Chamonix valley, where we spent so many glorious walking days; a painting of a Marabou stork; two Winnie the Pooh drawings; a lovely black and white photo of a primary school-aged boy and girl poring over a story book, maybe taken in the 60s; a photo postcard of a large Mandarin duck and a few of boats. We both loved boats. There's a photo of our first boat, Muriel 2, on the mooring, the swan family being fed off the stern, presumably sired by the swan we called Gregory, as he pecked. There's another of us in the cockpit which must have been taken by someone ahead of the mast, as it shows the sail caught tight and we are sailing along smiling. We were a good team, we learned how to sail together.

All these bits and pieces which, taken together, spoke to her of things she loved and were special. I cannot move them even though they are lopsided and curling at the edges.

Milestones in the Grief Observed

11 July 2008   Last week there were two hard milestones. Firstly, I had the taps in the bathroom changed back from the public loo type which (eventually) switch off on their own to normal ones. They are fine – I like them, but strangely it is telling me again that it's the end of an era. I was so relieved when I got those pressure-type taps as it meant I no longer had to get up several times a night to see if Irene had switched them off when she'd been out to the bathroom. She usually left them on, not a great disaster but annoying to wake up to no hot water. Secondly, I bought Irene some new trousers in her new size. Size 12. I could not believe they would fit her but they do. I bought her ones she would have liked. I can't bear to see her in old ladies' stretch things, so I bought her some trendy-looking jeans from Tesco's, two pairs. She is getting thinner. I feed her, almost force feeding, trying not to do what my mother did, which is to tell her I love her by feeding her, but it does make me feel better. Today I asked her if she missed me. I don't often make conversation as she cannot understand me anyway but I just wanted to ask her. I know the question is not fair. She heard the word miss, and she made a sentence with it in it, using it as Miss, maybe thinking about her school days. The other day she used several sentences with the word 'polo' in them, and I realised I was wearing my jacket with the word Polo on. I cannot imagine how her brain can still make sense of spelling.

I bought three books about loss and bereavement and grief, as if the answers might be in books. I don't think they will be, but it made me feel as though I am doing something. They were: *You'll Get Over It: The Rage of Bereavement* by Virginia Ironside, *In Loving Memory: A Collection for Memorial Services, Funerals and Just Getting By* edited by Sally Emerson, and *The New Black: Mourning, Melancholia and Depression* by Darian Leader. I also bought a book about Queen Victoria so that the cashier wouldn't think I was a total saddo, but actually I wanted to read more about her monumental mourning that I only know about from seeing the film *Mrs Brown*. It would seem that what she suffered from was melancholia, if by that we mean that the person who is left dies with the person who has actually died, whereas the mourner knows they are still alive, but they have to mourn and eventually they will stop mourning and feel better. But for the melancholic perhaps there is no happier time to come, and they are the ones who kill themselves out of grief or spend the rest of their lives not getting over it. I have befriended another woman whose husband is in the same care home. She says that when her husband dies she will want to throw herself into the grave with him. I could not feel more different. I want to live for the two of us, am desperate to live twice over; I want to get away from grief and misery. Does this mean I'm not a melancholic, but she is?

Yet what I have learned is that grief has its own pace. You cannot outwit it. I remember the most useful thing I learnt when I was starting to canoe – you can only control water if you go faster than it or slower than it. If you go at the same pace, the water has you in its control – you are not in control of it. Grief controls you; you can try to outwit it by rushing around to keep ahead of it, or you can lie low and pretend it's not happening, but grief catches up with you in the end.

15 July 2008   I found C S Lewis's book, *A Grief Observed*, and am reading it. It is so apt, written after his wife died, though there is nothing in the books which is similar to our situation – Irene is still alive. Ours is an ambiguous loss, I can see her, feel her, but she is not 'Irene'. The books on dementia and Alzheimer's presume that the sufferer is elderly and Irene is not; the books on losing relationships all assume that you are straight and also that you will perk up and start to find another man. I do not want anyone else, at least not right now. There is no single thing out there which matches my situation though I do find a huge solace in other people's tales of grief. It tells me that there is no way to circumnavigate the feelings – the grief work has to be done. You cannot take short cuts. I cannot believe how much better I feel after my mammoth cry-in on Sunday. I thought there would be no end to the tears. No, not just tears, big sobs from the very depths but now I feel like weight has shifted and I do feel happier. It will build up again of course. And there is still huge sadness, like not being able to tell you about all the little baby rabbits in the lane, or that the moon is almost full. I can only hold our previous life at arm's length or otherwise I would be overwhelmed by the sadness of the loss of it. But I do feel different after that good cry.

I picked up Lewis's book and the first paragraphs rang so true:

No one ever told me that grief felt so like fear. I am not afraid, but the sensation is like being afraid. The same fluttering in the stomach, the same restlessness, the yawning. I keep on swallowing.

At other times it feels like being mildly drunk, or concussed. There is a sort of invisible blanket between the world and me. I find it hard to take in what anyone says. Or perhaps, hard to want to take it in. It is so uninteresting. Yet I want the others to be about me. I dread the moments when the house is empty. If only they would talk to one another and not to me.

There are moments, most unexpectedly, when something inside tries to assure me that I didn't really mind so much, not so very much, after all. Love is not the whole of a man's live. I was happy before I ever met H. I've plenty of what are called resources. People get over these things. Come, I shan't do so badly. One is ashamed to listen to this voice but it seems for a little to be making out a good case. Then comes a sudden jab of red-hot memory and all this common sense vanishes like an ant in the mouth of a furnace.

Yes, it's like a switchback of self-delusion and self-pity; of sudden bouts of optimism and then overwhelming grief and sadness.

And no one told me about the laziness of grief. Except at my job – where the machine seems to run on much as usual – I loathe the slightest effort.

Yes, I can see that too. Last night after work – which does seem remarkably normal, I just sat, all evening really, and the evening sort of went by. I sorted out the old newspapers, and that was the extent of my activity. I feel better for having had a week pottering at home, and that was such a good decision not to go away. I would have been slogging up the A9 to John o'Groats if I hadn't come to my senses.

C S Lewis talks about how it doesn't matter where he goes – it's no worse if he goes to special places that he and his wife used to frequent, rather,

The act of living is different all through. Her absence is like the sky, spread over everything.

'Her absence is like the sky, spread over everything'. Irene's absence fills the house; it is getting bigger. Her absence fills all the cracks, seeps over all the surfaces, has its own life. Life is unutterably different, red where it was blue, dark where it was light, nothing remains the same.

And this separation, I suppose, waits for all. I have been thinking of H and myself as peculiarly unfortunate in being torn apart. But presumably all lovers are. She once said to me, 'Even if we both died at exactly at the same moment, as we lie here side by side, it would be just as much a separation as the one you're so afraid of.' Of course she didn't know, any more than I do. But she was near death; near enough to make a good shot. She used to quote Alone Into the Alone. She said it felt like that. And how immensely improbable that it should be otherwise! Time and space were the very things that brought us together, the telephone wires by which we communicated. Cut one off, or cut both off simultaneously. Either way, mustn't the conversation stop?

I cannot follow where Irene has gone; she has her own conversations and occasionally she does communicate with me and it is delightful. She is alive, though, but it feels a bit like she is dead to me. This is the conundrum of Alzheimer's. It is like nothing else. Even if someone went into persistent vegetative state, they would be closed to communication, not these sudden glimpses of the most eloquent phrases followed by gibberish.

16 July 2008   Irene seems to be getting thinner day by day. I read more of C S Lewis last night and he saw him and his wife as,

Two circles that touched. But those two circles, above all the point at which they touched, are the very thing I am mourning for, homesick for, famished for. You tell me she goes on. But my heart and body are crying out, come back, come back. Be a circle, touching my circle on the plane of Nature. But I know this is impossible. I know the thing I want is exactly the thing I can never get. The old life, the jokes, the drinks, the arguments, the lovemaking, the tiny, heart breaking commonplace… that is what we would all like. The happy past restored.

And the past is the past and that is what time means, and time itself is one more name for death, and Heaven itself is a state where the 'former things have passed away'.

I am dry-eyed at the moment. I am washed up, washed out. The tears have disappeared for the moment and I feel calmer.

The Cast

Irene now lives with a whole lot of other people, staff and residents. I know this is where she will be for the rest of her life. It seems strange to me, that she now lives with these people, all the time, people neither she nor I know, and with people who only know her as a person with dementia. They never knew her as she was. The staff do their best; they have personal photos on every residents' bedroom door, a montage of smiling family shots. I am getting to know the other residents, what I call 'the cast'.

Edna is either cheery or crying, and has a lilting Welsh accent. She sometimes talks in Welsh and always says to me 'I haven't seen you for a long time,' though I see her every few days. She put her hand on my face the other day and said, 'Oh, you have got such a lovely face, haven't you?' She often gets on her hands and crawls rather than using her walking frame. When I first met her she told me to stay on at school, not like her, leaving too early so having to work in a hairdresser's salon. She often says, 'Have you seen Fred?' Or, 'Have you seen my mother?'

George tries to muster people on to the parade ground. There's a picture of him, much younger, in an RAF uniform. The other day I had to call a nurse urgently as he was hauling the really infirm off their day beds. He often asks me if I'm coming along too: 'We're starting really early in the morning'. A feeling of *The Great Escape* comes over the ward and the more able are on some sort of secret alert. George has good speech and if we were not on a dementia ward you might think we were just exchanging pleasantries on the high street: 'Gloomy old morning!' sometimes delivered at dusk, or, 'Oh, there you are – been out?' He is concerned sometimes about the 'other chaps', especially when they are in a state of undress. 'This chap needs some help.' 'Well, not sure what's happening now.' He gives off a general air that things are not quite running properly but is a bit bemused about what can be done.

Jack is a strong good-looking older man, the sort who would build his grandchildren a tree house which would never blow down. He often talks about a wall he's building which needs more work, or how the car can't get down the drive because it's blocked, or all sorts of things which are going on in his head. The other night I watched as he put a cardboard box with a slipper inside into a sack like a pillow case, then wrapped it up in a blanket, then unwrapped it all, put a pair of shoes in, packed it up again like a knapsack, left it on a table, wandered off, came back, unpacked it all again with great deliberation, wandered off, came back to look for it. He is always polite and grateful if you point something out, like where he left his cap or bundle. He has an on/off relationship with George, the other day stopping him in a doorway and saying in a deliberate way, 'YOU hit me with that,' putting his strong hand on George's Zimmer, 'about a year ago.' And he glared at George in one of those male stand-offs which usually result in one backing off, which George did.

Marjorie was a headmistress. Her picture on the board outside her room shows a beaming younger women exuding efficiency and confidence, sure of her role. She now looks anxious and puffs around, not really making contact with anyone though looking fit-ish and occasionally joining in with George's conviction that the whole place has gone to the dogs and that they will shortly break out, using the number 36 bus.

Doreen has a picture of her receiving the MBE flanked by her two daughters. She was a star in the charity activities of Ripon. She now lies on her day bed, her body twisted like a dead bird's. Her daughter is a live bird, strutting about like a puffed-up pigeon. At first I thought she worked there, part of the hospitality staff, as she was so much on first-name terms with the residents and acted as if she belonged, handing out Maltesers. The staff seemed to see her as the relative from hell but actually she was very complimentary about them. The other day she cosied up to Barbara, trying to cajole her to get her lunch from the dining room. Barbara raised her hand as if to slap her and I thought 'good for you Barbara,' trying not to smile and pretending I hadn't seen the incident. Puffed-up pigeon moved her torso smartly back, and stepped away, her attempt at what the staff do totally rebuffed.

Barbara is a gentle woman, always dressed as if for an occasion, and talking very quietly in a mumbly, refined kind of way. She is one of the walkers, often on the move, loping in a lopsided way up and down the corridors.

Judy exudes disapproval, the sort of woman who would say to her insecure daughter, 'Are you going out like *that*?', knowing it would hit home and hurt. She stays in one chair, not being led to the dining room, perhaps because the staff know that she's better out there. Sometimes if she's in the mood she'll intentionally tip her dinner plate on to the floor, where it will land upside down and make a lovely mess. She is articulate and will say in a sharp voice, 'What are you doing that for?' as I, for example, help Irene with her food. I avoid her, try not to sit near her with Irene. On good days, she would have some lovely phrases, led by, 'That's disgusting!' or 'All these foreigners coming in'. These foreigners are the ones who look after her.

Vina is a Scot, another walker, pacing ceaselessly up and down and as a result as thin as a rake. The other day her daughter was keeping vigil by her bed as it seemed she was failing dramatically. Then to everyone's astonishment she was up and about again, her thin white face covered in blue bruises as if she had been hurled about in a washing machine.

Raymond takes up little space, sits in a chair and says in a wonderfully gravelly voice, 'I'm dying'. A few seconds elapse then: 'I'm dying…I'm dying…I'm dying'. He has his eyes closed. Sometimes he varies it by saying, 'I'm not well'. It's actually very funny as long as you don't let it get on your nerves.

Bill also has a lovely catch phrase, which is, 'Oh dear'. 'OH DEAR!' his voice rises as he is hoisted in the contraption which gets him out of his chair and into the wheelchair to take him back to his room. He tends to occupy the same chair in the day room, his round clown's face looking as if it's missing two large painted tears. He is short, with owlish glasses and only one leg. His entire leg is gone, the empty trouser neatly folded. His daughter looks just like him except she has all her limbs and, where he is bald, she has surprisingly big hair for a small person, but the same jolly disposition, a strong smile and quick movements. This genetic miracle applies to all the sons and daughters who look like their loved one, like in the opening scene of the original *101 Dalmatians*, where each dog resembles its owner (or the other way round).

Chris stands for long periods of time, his neck completely bent so that his gaze is fixed on the floor. And I know that he is the love of his wife's life, her beloved husband, so I look for him and check what he's doing. He is usually fairly comatose, sitting or standing and occasionally throwing out an expletive, 'Fuck off !' as someone lurches into him. Once he fell over just like David Jason at the bar in *Only Fools and Horses*. Sometimes he stands for an hour or more facing the wall like a praying monk.

Rita is another walker, lurching up and down the corridors and talking her own language, 'Doh doh doh doh, yes yes der der der der,' as she hurries on some errand. But she can also talk like a belligerent teenager, 'Well, I don't know, I went out and now I haven't got any, they've all gone, oh der der der der, and well I never said you could, so hop it! Yes HOP IT!' Hop it seems a favourite phrase and one that other residents understand, so they are always belligerent back. She is a furniture mover – she drags heavy chairs or cupboards down the corridor and is always immensely grateful and slightly surprised when the staff put food in front of her.

Adolf moves about and stares at you with quizzical eyes as if he can't quite place you. He sometimes copies behaviour, feeding Irene once with a pink biscuit, as that's what I was doing. I once asked him where he was from and, given his name, I thought he might just be old enough to be named for the Fuhrer. I said 'Germany?' 'No'. 'Hungary?' 'No'. 'Romania?' 'Yes,' with a slow smile dancing around his lips.

Shelagh has the eyes of a Bassett Hound. She is wonderfully Eeyore-ish and I once said to her 'Good morning,' and she replied , 'I doubt it'. She likes to be in her room, is egregious and looks slightly distrusting of everyone, staff included. She behaves as though she has woken up on another planet, which of course, she has.

These are the main characters, the ones who, if this was a film, would have some attention paid to them, have their character and history lingered over. The rest are the more shadowy ones, the ones who would cop it if there was a fireball or bomb, leaving the characters who we are really interested in to escape. I don't know their names. There are 30 or so residents, including Irene. They all are, or were, special to someone; were all once young, had active lives. They all have their histories, which they themselves have forgotten. They exist in the bubble of now.

And how would anyone sketch Irene? She is tall and thin, her head bowed over in a stoop. The result of drugs they say. She walks a lot and has a fixation for fire alarms and fire extinguishers. The fire brigade actually came once and it certainly perks up the staff, who all go on to red alert. Recently, each alarm has been covered in a Perspex case. She hoiks the large heavy extinguishers off their wall brackets and puts them on the floor or occasionally carries them a few yards, so they stand on the carpet like objects to be weaved around. And she needs help eating as she no longer can manipulate utensils. She sings and laughs and she smiles and waves energetically at any passing staff. She watches the other residents and makes contact with them, or sometimes seems to wonder what they are. She was Head of English at a secondary school and she is still so young. She has a partner called Rach who comes all the time. It's tragic.

An Inspector Calls

15 July 2008   Lovely visit to Irene today. She said straight away, 'I love, I love you, I love you,' and seemed so pleased to see me. She seemed brighter in herself unlike the other night when she was quite stroppy. It's amazing when she says that she loves me. Today she said she was frightened, a long word but I hope she wasn't frightened. She didn't seem so. There was a care home inspector who had called unannounced. She took me off to a corner and asked about activities and so on. I said Irene certainly couldn't take advantage of activities and what she needed was caring staff, which is what there is. Irene would not be aware of a singer who comes in to entertain, and anyway they seem to think that the songs the residents want to hear are 'Down at the Old Bull and Bush' rather than anything a bit more up to date. She asked me if I was a carer or a relative, which I thought an odd either/or question. I said a relative and only afterwards wished I'd said I was Irene's partner. Sometimes something in the person stops you coming out.

Afterwards I was talking to P and she said how she'd met a well-known actor on holiday and had kept in touch. When he lost his partner, P hadn't seen it like a marriage, but as losing his 'friend' and only now she wishes she had been more effusive in her regards to him after the bereavement. Many people do not see a gay relationship the same as a straight one, do not understand that how we love our partner is just the same as they love their husband or wife, that we are capable of such deep love for someone of the same sex. That's still the case with surveys into attitudes to homosexuality, that many do not see that civil partnerships are as significant or as meaningful as 'proper marriages'. It seems too, that people can pass the diversity training but cannot step outside a straight mindset.

I found out that the staff at the home were worried when they heard Irene had a female partner. It was new for them. I can't imagine what they were worried about but I am not prepared to ask. The wonderful manager took it as an opportunity to do some awareness training. We have only ever had courtesy, respect, and I get a sense of them really understanding what Irene and I were all about. It shows, I guess in how much we care for each other. And we did not go through the gay liberation battles of the 70s, 80s, and up to today, to go back into the closet when we are older. Being civil partners makes it easier. When asked I can just say, 'She's my civil partner,' or I can put that on a form. I have the legal right as next of kin. It makes me feel more secure. I've heard stories of the partner's family coming in, taking over, dispossessing a long-standing partner – not that anyone in our families would be like that.

I can honestly say I've had no bad experiences due to being in a same sex couple, with care services and so on. Things have moved on. The manager had been contacted by someone from Radio 4 to discuss experiences of being gay and in care. I agreed to be phoned by this journalist but she wasn't interested in our story as I'd only had good experiences and she wanted bad stories to tell, to expose the pockets of homophobia that do still exist. I asked her about balance but she wasn't interested.

Although I've not had bad experiences, it is true that I still, as all LGBT people do, make those judgments on the hoof about whether to come out, to be honest, or not. We should not have to do that, but we do. And it makes a huge difference to have people from the LGBT community running our services, like the relief manager, Micky, who I first felt so comfortable with at Irene's eventual choice of home, and with the manager who later returned to her post. It is such a relief simply to be understood.

I am convinced that the reason the consultant psychiatrist came out to our home, and that we had her, not the male (head) honcho, was because they assumed Irene had a problem with men. Neither of us do (some of our best friends are men!) but that was an assumption they made. The reason Irene had a problem with the head honcho was not because he was male but because he trod on her feelings like a hippo treading on orchids.

To Tell or Not to Tell?

11 July 2008   A friend was telling me about a friend of hers whose husband has been diagnosed with Alzheimer's and how he knows about it and they talk together about it. And I always feel a slight reproof, that I should have been more open with Irene. Maybe I feel it because I do indeed think I should have been more open, and now wish I had, that we had shared it all more. I wonder again how much of it was because I could not bear the pain of her pain of knowing. Knowing that she was losing the rest of her life, her happy 60s and that glorious slide into old age. Would she ever have come to terms with it? Was it better to pretend and cope as each day went along, until it was too late for her to comprehend anyway? I was on the brink of telling her so often, the pain of keeping it in like a physical pain, wondering at the time if it would alleviate what she was going through, that it would help her to understand. And often I wanted to do it in anger, when I was fed up with her behaviour, which obviously would have been the wrong thing to have done.

I can hardly bear to think about her knowing she was getting worse, that time she was upset about going to Spain to be with her good old university chums as she said, in tears, 'But I can't remember things'. What must she have gone through? It tears into me like a knife to think of it. To know of the suffering of your loved one and be able to do nothing. And I wonder if I did enough. I wonder if it was my inability to cope with it that meant I did not broach it. I told myself I was following Irene's lead, as she too did not seem to want to acknowledge the reality of it, but to live in a kind of denial.

Irene herself was told, I say to friends, defensively. We were both told on that dreadful day, by the consultant, that the most likely explanation was Alzheimer's but even by the time we were outside his room, Irene had not heard that word. She had an amazing ability to screen it all out. We had been to see Iris and she had been quiet and we both knew; so maybe she knew in her own way. She was ever the one to watch over me, just as I was the one to watch over her, and she was telling me in so many words that it was OK, we would survive this as our love for each other was the strongest thing in the world. Much later, she did see the word Alzheimer's on a leaflet left by the CPN and she said, 'Is that what they think I've got?', but by then she had gone into her happy-clappy stage, where she had no awareness of what she didn't know. That dreadful consciousness that things were not right had left her, and it was a happier time for us all. Small but significant losses were easier to bear, as she was not aware of them, like the last time she had to write her name on some form or other. I wrote it out for her and she copied it, as meekly as a child. I can see her name now, on a piece of paper on our kitchen table, in her handwriting, joined up letters gone, a signature saying who she was, though I'm not sure she knew what she had written.

Irene still has the wrist watch mark from last summer, a white band on her still-brown arms. I find it very moving, a sort of reminder. And another reminder – when we went down in the lift the other day, she saw herself in the mirror and she was delighted, exclaiming, 'It's me, it's me!' in exactly the same way she used to when she'd phone me up and say, 'It's me!' and I would be delighted. Especially if I was away and it was unexpected, but even if I was just at work it was lovely to hear from her, except of course later, when she'd phone me distressed, crying and obviously not coping. And I would not know what to do, torn between a work meeting or something, and thinking I should have been at home. How awful all that must have been, the mental torment. Thank God she is happy now. But all that horror preys on my mind. I have to find a way of dealing with it.

And the day-to-day reality of the dementia world carries on.

I went in to help Irene with lunch. There's a new resident called Margaret. She was curled up asleep in an armchair but every 30 seconds she said, 'I'm not getting up yet'. Sometimes she stressed the 'yet' and other times the 'up'. She sounded increasingly like a 15-year-old on a Saturday morning which had turned into the afternoon. Geraldine, one of the care workers, was trying to give her lunch, and she, Margaret, was increasingly resistant, saying and then shouting 'I don't want any more' but opening her mouth to receive it. Geraldine was coaxing her, saying she'd be hungry later. And I was getting agitated, as it reminded me of Irene shouting. I wanted to get away from the broken record (yes, it really was every 30 seconds, as I timed it), but, unusually for this week, Irene was very settled and wanted to stay put. All this week, she's been impossible to get to stay for a whole meal – she sits for a few minutes then gets up very determinedly to wander off. Anyway, I found myself saying to Margaret aloud what I'd meant to say to myself, which was, 'Oh shut up,' and it sounded just like my mother would have said it.

George came and sat next to Marjorie after lunch, and then wandered off, so another woman sat next to him. Then Marjorie came back and said, 'Oh sorry, am I intruding?' so George replied, 'No, this is just a friend of mine'.

Irene was her happy self, talking a lot today. She says whole sentences but they don't relate to anything I can see. Or she'll start a sentence but it will end in mumbles so I never quite catch what she might be intending to say. She might say, 'Yes well that's what I think and then, she stooped down and [mumble mumble]'.

Kitty was standing leaning with her arms outstretched on either arm of the chair in which Adolf was sitting, pinning him in. She said, 'Can you take me to the hospital because I need to see my grandmother – she's there, you see. Do you know Croker Street in Workington?' Adolf, from Romania, looked straight at her but said nothing. 'You see, she says "I want to see my little Kitty, my little Kitty," and I need to get home before my dad does; she always wants to see her little Kitty, that's me you see and I need to get the things for our tea and my grandmother isn't well, not well at all …' and she carried on in this vein for some time. Kitty was looking out the window and saying how lovely the green lawns were, how very green. Finally Adolf, tired of being bemused, wandered over to me and said, 'She likes looking outside,' in his strong eastern European accent. Kitty is in her eighties I would think and so small it's a wonder she finds women's clothes rather than those for a child.

And I wonder if what happens when people get dementia is that the essence of what they are gets distilled, all other things about them stripped away. What's left is something true about them – Irene seems happy; by all accounts she was a happy smiley baby. Those who are angry now, or disappointed, or raging, or resigned, or kindly – maybe that is what's there in the real core of their being. That bit of personality which seems to pop out of the womb, and is a constant. Maybe that's what it comes down to now.

A Major Case of Chattering Classes Angst

22 July 2008   There is a lovely sunset, the sky soft pinks and greys, and you would have shrieked in delight and called me to see it –'Ooh, come and look at the sky!', and I would have.

The wormery has arrived, part of my on-going spending spree. I never understood retail therapy till now. I fitted it together, which we would have enjoyed once, doing it together. Anyway, it promises to transform the garden, creating lush growth out of worm pee. I also bought a new lawnmower and, as usual with my purchases made without consultation, I have probably bought the wrong one. It is too heavy. I went for a good reliable one and it weighs a ton. You would have talked me out of it. And I miss the old Mountfield, which we'd had for over 20 years, and I miss having something which you had handled. Also it doesn't make the lawn look any better, which is what I thought it would do. Maybe it's my mowing technique. That was always your job, though we never really paid it much attention, often leaving it till it looked like a field, out of place in our village of anal lawn scalpers who make their lawns look like the serving ends at Wimbledon at the end of the tournament. Anyway, the Mountfield has gone and I am left with a large Hayter which runs away with me.

I am now worried about my heart. I saw the GP about suspected asthma and I thought, 'That's what it was, this tightness in my chest'. He asked if it was there all the time and I said I didn't think so, and he said, 'Because, of course, the other thing it could be is your heart'. I dismissed it at the time but now I'm worried. Can you look after someone with Alzheimer's for over five years and not get a dicky heart? Joan, who looked after her increasingly violent husband, had a minor heart attack when he went into care, but she was in her sixties. I'm only 54. I keep wondering and listening and the tightness does seem to be slightly more on the left side. I don't know what to think. I spent the relaxation time at yoga drooling about buying a bag of

109

chips on the way home, but instead went and bought six organic free-range eggs.

Yesterday I saw my counsellor and I told her I was in the middle of a yawning fit. She said that some people say yawning is a releasing suppressed anger. I said I thought it was because I was shattered. I have been wondering whether I would feel anger at some point but really all I feel is sad. Should I feel angry? I'm worried now that I have suppressed anger; maybe that's why I have a tight chest.

Darian Leader in his book on melancholia and grief writes: 'Absence is never accepted without rage', and 'Rage is ubiquitous in the mental life of bereaved people'. Later he says we 'can feel fury without being consciously aware of it'. Confusing or what? I did feel enormous fury earlier, like when we had spent a week or so walking in Devon, and I went berserk, so much so that I broke a good strong Leki walking pole, as I'd hit it so many times against the grass bank we were walking beside. Later I sobbed out loud further along the country lane, out of Irene's hearing, howling in rage.

Has it all gone? Or will I rage again when Irene dies? For I have not been bereaved in the conventional sense, not had to deal with her death. I am not conscious of anger or rage, just profound sadness. I did have that ambivalence before, which comes from love being close to hate. There were times I thought the only way out was to kill Irene, and I rationally contemplated this; smothering her seeming the easiest way. I went into a kind of madness, maybe a year and a half ago, when I was in the thick of it. I hated her at times, hated what our life had become, hated what she took out of me, hated the inequality that had become so part of our relationship, me now a carer. Hated her, really. I once went up to my study and wrote out 'That it's come to this' hundreds of times on paper. That our special partnership had been so wrecked by a bloody awful disease. All that has gone too, and I only feel love, sadness, enormous pity and I just want to say, oh my poor one, my special one, where have you gone, and why?

Yesterday you said to me, 'I'm proud of you,' and I have to stop myself believing that somehow you know. It's hard when at other times you say things like, 'John, John, we need to get out and ...' Then unintelligible. How can I believe that one thing makes sense and not another? We don't know anyone close called John but you do use that name a lot. But I want to believe that you are proud of me, and

I know that when you say, 'I love you' it means that you do love me. I know this.

I miss you. I miss you so much.

There's a lot in the papers about the Lambeth conference and gay people not being bishops. The ordained gay American bishop, Gene Robinson, said in a sermon that fear is the opposite of love, not hate, and I think he's right. Fear of the Other. Those people who are so fearful of we who love each other. I bet they cannot imagine the depth of love we are capable of feeling for each other. Desmond Tutu has said that surely the church has more to be concerned about – poverty, climate change, AIDS – whereas it seems obsessed with homosexuality. In my naivety I think that surely if they understood my love for Irene, they would be OK about it, but I guess that's not the point.

27 July 2008   There was a piece in the *Observer* today, one of those slightly self-indulgent, middle-aged, middle-class angst pieces about an aspect of lifestyle, which happened to be on memory. Each generation seems to discover that it can't remember quite as well as it used to, and the chattering classes respond by writing about it. Much of it was irritating but he did say this well:

Memory isn't just something, it's everything – the sum of who we are, the glue, page and spine of our story, the repository of our identity. It's no more than a handful of sludge but it's also vast – a great galaxy of all we have experienced and known, constantly updating, drawing meaning from the absurd blizzard of life to make and shape and sharpen our personalities and intellects and feelings.   (Phil Hogan, 27 July 2008)

You always explained your illness to others by reaching up to your neck and saying you had 'this problem at the back of my neck', and indeed our most simple memories are stored at the back of our brain, in the neural circuitry that is in the visual cortex near to where you would point. I can see you now, with your hand cupping the back of your neck. Where am I in the neurons of your brain? The science would say I am near the front, in the temporal lobes, where the more complicated memories are stored, maybe a scattering of neurons which tell you that I am me, and you are you, and let you still say your name, Irene Heron, which you do from time to time. The scan of your brain must have been pretty conclusive to the consultant, your brain already shrunken, showing the irreversible loss of neurons. The sludge that is our brain had become, in your case, something that looked wrong and the only explanation was Alzheimer's.

A few months ago I said to my counsellor that I needed a marker, something significant to show that our relationship was lost. It is not a divorce, not a death; you are still there but so very not here. What ceremony can help? If I was angry with an unfaithful partner I might burn your things, or if you had died I would have your ashes and I would do something special with them. I said what I thought I'd do is take some things of yours and put them in Windermere. But now this seems wrong. I imagined a capsule of things, maybe a photo, I don't know. And I would sink it in the deep part of the lake where it could never be found. Now I find this gloomy and melodramatic and also I don't like the thought of you – pieces of your life – down there in the cold deep. So I will not do that. It seems more poignant and more positive to take the canoe out and enjoy the lake you loved so much.

And it is slowly getting into my head that our relationship is not here any more; it is there still of course, a huge collection of memories of a shared life and an effect on me that has made me what I am, but it will now always be in the past; it is not going anywhere, not still growing. And the sadness sits on my shoulders – what fun we would have had! Still climbing mountains, walking along beaches, stopping at pubs for a half pint of shandy and a packet of crisps, our formula for a good time. You sometimes would point to an elderly pair of women walking along the street and say, 'That will be us one day,' and already I knew then that it wouldn't be, me privy to knowledge you never did acquire, that we would not grow old together as we wanted.

Losing what the person was but not losing the person – anyone with a relative or partner with dementia or a personality change or mental illness must experience this. But how do you mourn it?

You look at me with those same grey-blue eyes.

And waking up in the night I stretch out my arm and remember how you would be there, and I would turn and snuggle up to your back, a simple pleasure and a joy.

As I was leaving you the other day, my new chum from the care home suddenly said 'It does get better you know'; she no longer thinks about her husband as soon as she wakes up and has times when she doesn't have him at the surface of her mind. It's been three and half years since he was admitted, and this has just started to happen. I silently bless her for telling me this, knowing I cannot say anything or I will cry.

3 August 2008   There's a piece in the paper (*Guardian* 2 August 2008) today about a new way to treat dementia, billed as 'a revolution in dementia care'. Basically, Penny Garner has argued that dementia sufferers need to have their reality understood and then their behaviour makes sense. As people lose their short-term memory they rely on their older memories and use these to make sense of their present. As they have no idea of who they might be talking to or where they are, they get aggressive and behaviour becomes unmanageable (tell me about it!), and so they are prescribed anti-psychotic drugs as this is the only way carers can cope. But if you understand that person's reality, you can use it to organise their routine etc. As John Cleese might say, seems 'bleedin' obvious' to me.

It also criticises anti-psychotics, which 'dope, befuddle and reduce communication'. It seems people have been helped to come off medication and in some cases live at home again. Whew. It's hard seeing things like this, as it always makes me feel guilty. Am I doing the right thing for Irene? Did we do the right thing getting her admitted? Why did she go downhill so quickly after she started on the anti psychotics? The other day her main nurse and the manager were trying to explain about what happens if someone stay on the drugs after they don't really need them and also what happens if someone comes off them. It seemed that if they come off they can deteriorate rapidly and if they can stay on…they can also deteriorate rapidly…how on earth can we make a decision?

The book is called *Contented Dementia: 24 hour Wrap-around Care for Life-long Well-being* by Oliver James. Any revolution feels too late for Irene. It makes me ache thinking about it, the ache of being too late. This is the biggest angst of all, not knowing if I am doing the right thing, Irene's care entrusted to me – well, not really, as the professionals make the decisions but …

'Contented dementia' indeed!

Before that, Irene's specialist had called, a Dr B – she's a psychiatrist, I guess, and she seemed very nice. I have not spoken to any doctor about Irene's medication since 2007, (or early 2008?) so this was timely. She is wondering about halving the Amilsulpride, which is the drug which causes the neck to droop. It's hard to know what to do, so I said to try it and see. The anti-dementia drug Irene is on is Galatamine, which she might as well stay on. The other is the anti-psychotic, which some reports are saying should not be used for dementia anyway. But they routinely are. What do you do when someone is frightened and aggressive because they are deluded? Talk them out of it? The other night I sat up in bed and thought, 'I do not know' – i.e. how to treat Irene or whether her drugs should be reduced or what, and I felt better . Why had I been trying to puzzle it out? How can I be expected to know?

Today Irene was in a good mood, kicking up one leg in a funny gesture when we were walking outside. I realise that I measure how good my visits are by whether she said anything nice to me, which means that she recognizes who I am, that she loves me; by whether she is alert and happy; by how much food I can get down her.

An Evening at the Bishop's

5 August 2008 My counsellor talks about a time of crisis being a time when you can recreate yourself any way you want, and it's true that I have found myself in situations of which I would otherwise have said, 'No, that's not quite our thing.' Take that party at Chrissie's where there was a group doing Tibetan nose singing. I chickened-out of the follow-up, a night of mole charming at a quarry where we were encouraged to bring tents for overnight stays, and also told not to wear moleskin trousers in case it upset the moles. Anyway, last night was the other extreme, a fundraiser at the Bishop of Ripon and Leeds' house near Ripon. It was large enough to house about 200 Africans. The Bishop himself was off at the synod but his wife was an archetypal bishop's wife (not that I'd met one before). I tried to mention the Archbishop of York's welcome common sense that they had more important things to talk about than gay priests but I think she was too preoccupied with having 75-plus members of the great and good of Harrogate and Ripon society in her house. These were the sorts of people with prominent Yorkshire accents, so a little status-insecure, who are quite wealthy and would be absolutely delighted to have their photo taken with minor aristocracy or even better, any royal, and then get it into *Yorkshire Life*. It was a wine tasting followed by an auction of promises. We had 13 wines and, not being much of a drinker, I have to admit I pigged out on the food which was meant to accompany them and which was delicious. I notice they whipped it all away during the auction, as some of us had already eaten.

£10-worth plus the wine. Anyway, I bid for a day of windsurfing lessons for

£90. I meant to stop at £80 – someone else's bid – but then thought what the hell, I've always wanted to learn to windsurf. And it's for a good cause.

It was all terribly middle class and terribly straight. There was a flautist playing in one of the reception rooms. Each room was large enough to be a reasonable-sized bedsit. The huge staircase was filled with life-size portraits of previous bishops. It's the last event which will be held there as Bishop and household are moving to Leeds, which is where most of the diocese live. I wondered if Bishop and wife would move to Seacroft or Beeston or any of the other centres of deprivation, but I suspect they won't.

My chums dropped me at home. And as I walked up the stairs I felt that fleeting disappointment – again – that Irene is not here. The darkness in the house was sort of comforting but also told me I was alone. I didn't know what else to do but go to bed. Normally we would have the recounting of the evening, discussing who we'd seen, what had happened, laughing. Instead I had just myself, and as I had relaxed, I had momentarily forgotten that Irene would not be here. It still feels so normal for her to be here, at the end of a day, the person I would check in with, my anchor.

An evening where I was reminded of other worlds, the world that is normal for some, the Bishop's house, the world of wealth and middle-classness in leafy Ripon. The house is hidden from the road, just a sign telling you it is there, so no one would normally see it. And Irene's place is the same, a sign off the road to a large building where most people would never stray, and a closed world inside, a world that is the centre of the world for those living there, the only world. None of these worlds is more real than any other. I glimpse them all but feel really at home in none.

And it still surprises me that I have not fully taken it in that Irene now is elsewhere, after she has been gone for almost a year. I guess 11 months after nearly 27 years of her being here is a small proportion, and also my heart wants her to be here. I still sometimes think, 'OK, let's go back to normal now, I've had enough of this,' as though you're playing hide and seek and you get fed up of looking – OK, this has gone on for long enough, come out now.

The End of a Year of Magical Thinking

4 August 2008   It's coming up to a whole year since Irene went into care.

I am scared of forgetting and scared of remembering. There are things I don't want to think about and things I am worried that I cannot remember, like now remembering why Irene's behaviour was so awful. I do not want to lose any part of her but my subconscious seems to have blocked some of it out. I remember the feelings – of drawing up in the car outside the house and feeling I could not face going in, of curling up in a foetal position in a corner where I could not easily be found, of waiting for the verbal blows. I remember her getting up in the morning and hitting her angry stride, furious that the clothes she wore yesterday (and the day before) were not there. And she would come to my side of the bed where I was hoping to doze and shout at me that she had nothing to wear. I would say something placatory and she would shout something like, 'Don't you care that I've nothing to wear?' I would get up and try to find her something that would do. She would storm off and then come back – and so it would go on. And sometimes I would get angry too.

Maybe then she would say that she would get me a cup of tea so she would go down to the kitchen and then forget. I would tiptoe down to see where she was, and then she'd feel bad, having forgotten. Then she would maybe bring me two cups, one after the other, and be furious that I was already drinking one, as she couldn't remember having brought me it. And I would feel worn out before I'd even got up. Then she would come and sit on the edge of the bed and cry, and say how useless she was, and I would say, 'No you're not!' and hug her. But we both knew it was no good.

And the constant need she had to be with me, so I could not do anything without her demanding I was with her. I'd try to make a phone call or check my email and within a minute or so she would be there, saying the TV had gone off, and she didn't know how to get it back, or she couldn't change channel, or the fire was going out and could I come? And I'd say yes, just a minute, and then she'd be back in a few seconds. I learnt how to do Sudoku as it's one of the few activities you can do in the few seconds while the one with dementia is distracted; it can be dropped and come back to, needing only short bursts of concentration. I remember her storming out of umpteen restaurants if the food wasn't quite what she thought it was going to be.

I'm sorry. Did I do all I could? Did I manage it properly? Was I partly to blame for how you behaved? It's too hard to remember; I want to forget but I cannot forget, don't want to forget. Memories. And I had to face every day living with the knowledge I was losing her without being able to share any of that losing with her. Losing the most precious thing and wanting to cry but not being able to let her know – the one person I told everything else to. How did I cope with all that?

I was talking about all this with my counsellor. I said trying to remember is like trying to hold on to jelly, or frog-spawn, or water. It trickles through your hands with an energy of its own. I feel I have no control over it. And later I thought about how she has been on this journey with me. I've been so lucky to have found a good counsellor, had the gumption to realise I needed it, and had the money to pay for it. Darian Leader says: 'Without some form of third party, we have no anchor, no way of believing in the authenticity of what we have been through.' He talks about how someone going through a loss will seek out such a third party in order to play this authenticating function. He mentions the case of a woman, who had lost her mother, having a dream where she was telling a faceless stranger all about it. 'By introducing a basic triangulation, it showed that the loss was being registered, transformed into a message to be transmitted to someone else and accepted, at some level, by herself.'

Basically, this seems a convoluted and clever way of saying that we need someone to talk to, and when we find that someone it makes it all real. I could not have done this mourning without my fortnightly counselling. And telling this story, which has become one I am relating to an audience, I am also making it real. If someone listens to us, it must be real. I know that I really only ever know what I feel when I hear what I say. But it's so hard to get the words out.

But how I wish I could take a tranquillizer and wake up and it would all be over! Everyone says you have to do the grief work, there are no short cuts. Just grit your teeth and get through it, and believe, really believe, that time is the great healer. And the other benefit of counselling, and the reason I have stuck with it, is that I didn't want to get to the very end (what do I mean –Irene's death?) and then have to start to deal with it. I wanted to get the account up to date as I went along – no backlog. It feels that life is too short to wait to get over this. A decade of dementia and then a decade of coming to terms with it, sorting it all out in my head? No thank you! I will have a life to get on with. Anyway, I also needed a wise counsellor just to keep me going.

I don't know what I want. Everything seems empty, and I am making things up to fill in the time, time without you, and towards the time when I won't feel this bad. I have all sorts of little projects, routes I want to walk, things I want to do in the garden, but really I am making up things to do. There seems to be so much time now you're not here. In the past time was never a problem, before you were ill. We were always just occupied if the other was around. Chatting about things or just being quiet together.

Tomorrow a guy is coming to replace the two little broken panes of glass which shattered when you were in a temper and slammed the hall door. They have been stuck with tape for over a year. It's not the first time they have had to be mended; I've shattered them myself before. Maybe we two should never have had doors with glass panes.

5 August 2008   You looked at me today with those same adoring eyes that made me realise you loved me, back in 1980, sitting on the floor at a party. I was on a chair and you were on the floor, and I thought, alarmed and delighted, 'Crikey! She loves me'. I wept today, and you saw I was crying, and you held my hands. I can't bear seeing you like this, demented, away from me, walking up and down in a care home. You look at me sometimes as if you know who I am but can't quite place me. Later you said, 'Because I love you,' and you read two words, 'critical test', in the paper, headlines about Kevin Pietersen taking over as England cricket captain. The lunch was late, as there had been a practice evacuation (said Jeanette, rolling her eyes heavenwards). And I fed you two plates of lunch and two puddings.

Every day is an anniversary, the first. I am going over all the things we have lost, all the fun we would have had, in this first summer without you. The first August where we have not had plans together. I long to do the things we used to, to walk in the Alps from hut to hut, that wonderful feeling of exploration. Now I am unfit and mentally exhausted, and I don't see the point of going anywhere on my own or even with anyone else. We had the whole of the rest of our lives to enjoy doing things in each other's company. And we lost it. We lost it.

Grief feels like the layers of an onion – you think you are peeling a layer away to get to the other side of something where it's better but instead you just go deeper into the misery. You start all over again at a deeper layer. It's hard to believe it's still all there, as fresh as ever. Seeing you at times is unbearable and not seeing you is unbearable too. We were together today, you comforting me in a way that I think you knew you were doing, a tiny spark of recognition.

6 August 2008　　　　I'm not seeing Irene today, though I could, and I have the time. I can't face another day of emotional turmoil. I'm worried that if I'm not there she won't get enough to eat but I just need a day to myself. I feel like Irene and I used to feel sometimes returning after some heroic feat of endurance, and all you want to do is sit and watch the laundry go round in the washing machine. I have come to a standstill, exhausted.

Yesterday I sorted out some of Irene's clothes, the ones I know will not be needed (too big) and not be right for me (too small). Most went happily into the black bin liners but then I uncovered your first fleece, that pink and grey one which you wore so much and was so 'you'. And I clutched it to my face and wept. It's back in the wardrobe. I still find it so hard to think of you not coming back as you were then, full of life and energy. There's something you made when you were in primary school, which hangs on the wall of the room I'm in now, your old study, and it says 'Glad that I live am I, that the sky is blue'. It's in your child's handwriting with a painted border. It's one of the things I'd save if the house were on fire.

7 August 2008　　　　　When I went to see about my trapped nerve, the physio asked if I lived alone, and I said through clenched teeth, 'Yes', feeling quiet resentment filling my head, and wanting to say, 'But I've had a very successful and happy relationship for nearly 30 years, and it was only cut short by illness. I AM A SUCCESSFUL HUMAN BEING! I AM NOT A FAILURE!!' Because that's what I realise I feel like. A failure. I have not managed to keep a life-long marriage, one that slipped into comfortable old age.

The innings are over but I wasn't out. I stayed in; it was the game that ended.

I do not like having to reconstruct myself and I do not like the lie that I am single.

In the space where I am, caught between not being able to remember and not being able to forget, I read this, written by Freud: 'We will never find a substitute [after a loss]. No matter what may fill the gap, even if it be filled completely, it nevertheless remains something else. And actually, this is how it should be, it is the only way of perpetuating that love which we do not want to relinquish'. And that makes a lot of sense – I do not want to lose anything, let go of anything, yet I also want this terrible, unbearable grief to be over, and I want to be happy, and maybe even be loved, and love, someone else.

The cliché that losses need to be worked through so that we can move beyond them suggests that mourning is something that can be done and dusted. We are encouraged so often to 'get over' a loss, yet bereaved people and those who have experienced tragic losses know full well it is less a question of getting over a loss and on with life, than finding a way to make that loss part of one's life Darian Leader.

It's sunny – I'm going outside.

9 August 2008   So I suppose the work of mourning is a bit like building a garden – it's never really finished, there's always a bit more to do, even if you're happy with it.

Someone yesterday told me it was the luckiest occasion in history – the 8th minute of the 8th hour of 8th day of the 8th month, in the year 2008. I slept through it. I think I had gone back to sleep, the alarm rousing me at 8.15.

At 7.20 in the morning the phone had rung. I was fast sleep. It was Pam from Irene's home. She said Irene had had a fit and had also a bump, as she'd fallen. I mumbled thanks for letting me know. The previous night she had been not very well when I saw her, for once not wanting chocolate. She actually said, 'I feel sick'.

The whole of my family who live close to me is about to decamp to the other side of the world. I'm dealing with so much stuff.

The borough council sent a letter asking if Irene was still severely mentally impaired and if she still lived here. I wrote to say she was no longer here, the words in black type telling the truth. This was one of the things I wish social services had told me earlier, as it saves me £1,000 per year. I can't remember how I found out that you get reduced council tax if you live alone, but it wasn't social services that told me… Anyway I will still get reduced rates, as I am now the sole occupant. The sole occupant.

The sole occupant of our house, and the silence and the space are enormous. But you are here too, in your things and in the memories and in your spirit, the fact you were here; you were here, that is true and real, and even if you will not be here again, you were here.

31 August 2008   I've been in Italy on my holiday and it was only after 29 August had passed that I remembered the anniversary I was dreading. I had the first really relaxing holiday for about eight years. I have thought through whether I'm exaggerating – is this really the first relaxing holiday in so long? Really, it was. But I was 20 minutes from getting off the train to the airport to come home when I was hit by a really clever scam: tap on the shoulder in the train, turned round, looked back after literally five seconds and my rucksack with everything in it – hand luggage – had gone. Passport, money, bank cards, two cameras, my beloved 11 x 50 Optolyth binocs, sunglasses, iPod, other bits and pieces, including the lovely blue pullover jacket that I love and which used to be Irene's. The luggage was on the window side and I was in the aisle seat so the accomplice must have reached over me as I turned. I didn't even register until the train was pulling out of the station. The polizia say it happens every day at Trastevere station. So why the f*** don't they do anything about it? I knew at once the rucksack was gone.

I got on the flight OK and now am home; amazing how you can cross borders when you are articulate and white, with absolutely no papers or ID. Maybe being female and middle-aged helps too. I felt oddly liberated in Rome airport, no heavy hand luggage, literally relieved of my baggage. Somehow I can't get too upset. I think it's because compared with what I have lost, it's like comparing the size of a rucksack to the size of the moon. And everything there is replaceable. Also I felt certainty – I knew I would never see my stuff again. It was certain – I could from that moment, start to get over it. It's uncertainty that I can't cope with. I realise that it's the uncertainty of the last however many years – eight? – that is so wearing. The uncertainty of whether it's Alzheimer's or not? How fast will she decline? Should we be thinking about extra help? Uncertainty all the time. It's one of the things that makes dementia so wearing; you live with the jitteriness of uncertainty, jumping around like someone on a caffeine high.

My sister said she went to see Irene, and as she was feeding her some chocolate. Penny shed a tear, and Irene put her hand up and wiped it away. It's hard coming back to this. I cried too when I saw Irene. It was so great being away, being warm, lovely blue skies, no worries. Sometimes I realised I hadn't thought about Irene for a whole day. I feel weary about facing it all again.

18 September 2008 It's been a year since Irene left. I have only just started going into the living room again in the evenings, the warm heart of our home, you sitting at one end of the settee and me at the other. You would say, 'Put something jolly on!', and I would choose Rossini as that's what you thought was jolly. And you would be knitting and I would be reading the paper. And all would seem right with the world.

I have just finished reading Joan Didion's book *The Year of Magical Thinking*, a reflection of the year after her husband of 40 years, John, died suddenly from a major heart attack. Although it is so different from my experience – hers the sudden and dramatic exit of her loved one, shockingly abrupt heartbreak, and mine the slow, tortuous heartbreaking every day all over again – she has a lot to say about grief and the whole awful business of it.

Something she writes speaks to me as I've been in the last few weeks, struggling to find meaning without Irene:

Grief turns out to be a place none of us know until we reach it. We anticipate (we know) that someone close to us could die, but we do not look beyond the few days or weeks that immediately follow such an imagined death. We misconstrue the nature of even those few days or weeks. We might expect that if death is sudden to feel shock. We do not expect this shock to be obliterative, dislocating to both body and mind. We might expect that we will be prostrate, inconsolable, crazy with loss. We do not expect to be literally crazy, cool customers who believe that their husband is about to return and need his shoes. In the version of grief we imagine, the model will be 'healing'. A certain forward movement will prevail. The worst days will be the earliest days. We imagine that the moment to most severely test us will be the funeral, after which this hypothetical healing will take place. When we anticipate the funeral we wonder about failing to get through it, rise to the occasion, exhibit the strength that invariably gets mentioned as the correct response to death. We anticipate needing to steel ourselves for the moment: will I be able to greet people, will I be able to leave the scene, will I even be able to get dressed that day? We have no way of knowing that the funeral itself will be anodyne, a kind of narcotic regression in which we are wrapped in the care of others and the gravity and meaning of the occasion. Nor can we know ahead of the fact (and here lies the difference between grief as we imagine it and grief as it is) the unending absence that follows, the void, the very opposite of meaning, the relentless succession of moments during which we will confront the experience of meaninglessness itself.

I am in the void, the relentless knowing that you are not here, that this is how it will be. For ever and ever. Yet when I have seen you, twice recently, you managed to bring out from somewhere in your damaged brain, 'I want, want to see, see you' and another day, straight away, 'I love you'. And it is me that you love, so I feel terrible not being there, and wondering if you're wondering where I am. How can you still say those things yet be so demented at other times? It only occurred to me the other day that, just as I know so well, your every gesture, your walk, that I know the back of your head better than you do. And you will have known my every look and gesture, the back of my head, and that must all still be imprinted in your mind somewhere.

I think too that maybe you'll come back, like the other day at the barbecue when I heard someone and I didn't think, 'That sounds like Irene'. I thought 'That's Irene' and I turned, and of course it wasn't.

'I cannot count the days on which I found myself driving abruptly blinded by tears'. Yes and every song on the car radio speaks to you, and brings the tears on. '…But I miss you most of all my darling when autumn leaves start to fall'. 'You are the sunshine of my life'. Joan Didion quotes Phillippe Aries: 'A single person is missing for you, and the whole world is empty…But one no longer has the right to say so out loud.'

She repeats throughout the book: 'Life changes fast. Life changes in an instant. You sit down to dinner and life as you know it ends.' I feel the opposite. Life has changed imperceptibly, so slowly that I can't figure out when it began to change, and it's been going on for so long I can't remember what life was like before. I do not understand the concept of a normal life, a life which did not revolve around Irene's needs. I am realising that it started long before I saw it happening. I am reading Graham Stoker's book of stories from his clinical experience of people with dementia. The small signs that relatives began to act on were all there with Irene too.

Joan Didion adds to her mantra 'The question of self pity'. We worry, she says, about wallowing in it – what's the right level of grief? What can we display and what should we keep to ourselves? Gloria Hunniford was interviewed yesterday about the death of her daughter, and she was asked by the *Woman's Hour* presenter to sum up, and she said: 'Well, you can cry all you like but it won't bring them back so you might as well get on with it.' How sorry for ourselves should we feel? Recently I've begun to feel resentful of what I've been robbed of and what awful circumstances Irene has ended up in. She should be out walking, enjoying retirement like our friends are. Instead she is with people a generation older than she is, walking the corridors, shut off from ordinary life. We both had so much ahead of us, so much we could have done. I resent this deeply. We woz robbed!

The other day Linda told me that they went in to get Irene up and somehow she had managed to work the control which pumps her bed up and down and she was six feet off the floor, 'Her little eyes peeping over the bed'. It was funny and sad.

Joan Didion says that the bereaved forget to breathe. I go around holding my breath too. Anyway I am sleeping better, which helps. Robins are singing their autumn song, there's a nip in the air and it feels as though the change of season is on its way. She finishes her book by talking about how they used to go to a certain cave, swimming in from the sea, and how John taught her how to wait and watch for exactly the right moment, to feel the swell change, and how to catch it.

And I know I'm a subtly different person who came back from Italy, so change is happening.

I have a new passport, using the fast track service. I went to see *Mamma Mia* (for the third time) while I waited for my new identity to emerge.

Irene still squeezes my knees when I see her. Last night she put her legs up across mine, like she used to.

Darian Leader writes:

We have explored four processes which signal that the work of mourning is taking place: the introduction of a frame to mark out a symbolic, artificial space, the necessity of killing the dead, the constitution of the object – involving the separation of the image of the loved one and the place they occupied for us – and the giving up of the image of who we were for them.

I wish he would write in more accessible English, but I think I know what these words mean. Firstly it seems to be about marking out your own space. I have a recurring fantasy about wanting to buy a small cottage, near the sea, where I can be myself. Secondly, I realise I need to move forwards, not 'killing' Irene but distinguishing myself from her. She was my life. That's all I wanted. Who am I now? Thirdly I need to start seeing her as her, and not just as my partner with all that that involved. Fourthly, I need to give up being the faithful and adoring partner.

Do I really?

PART THREE:
ENDINGS AND BEGINNINGS

My Poor Love

10 February 2009   Irene's birthday

A friend sends Irene a card: 'Make a birthday wish', it says on the front, and inside, 'Hope they all come true'.

I want to throw it in the bin. So I do.

13 February 2009   I haven't written for so long. I am sick at heart. My poor love. You broke your ankle, we're not sure how. I am where? On the scale of things? I miss you so much that I've started to fantasize about what you might have been like, now at 62, a wonderful person who loved me – and we did have a special love, didn't we? Please tell me we did. Please tell me you love me, one more time. I don't think you ever will again because you have stopped saying anything like that, the words are all gobbledygook now. I am alone and I feel lonely. Too late to come and see you tonight.

22 February 2009   I dreamed that we were in bed and Irene was kind of over on my side, diagonally across the bed, so I was scrunched up against a wall. I couldn't get her to understand to move over and I had to extricate myself from her hug to get out of bed. I went out of the room, which was a hotel kind of room, around a very large courtyard. My mother was out there and there was a guy mowing the lawn. We said why are you doing this now, in the middle of the night when we want to sleep, and he said, well, there's so much lawn to mow, I have to do that bit now. My mother and I both remonstrated with him. I wanted to find another room to sleep in as I couldn't get any rest in the same bed as Irene – she took up all the room.

 When I saw my counsellor she asked me what I thought the dream was about and I said I thought it was fairly obvious. I needed more space, I needed quiet and my mother, dead these past five years, was there backing me up. That is how I feel.

I cannot believe how hard this still is. I feel tormented by not having Irene in my life and knowing that this is how it will be. Seeing her is torture too, my poor love. So much that she has lost; all right for me – I've lost her, us, but I have everything else. She has lost it all. She doesn't know it, thank God. But other 62-year-olds are out there still being young.

Easter 2009   And what of memory? I want memories, just to remember. So much forgetting, I want to remember it all, urgently, as if I am the one with the impaired memory. All memory is impaired in that memory isn't a faithful rendition of what was. Funny how Irene could remember some things which I couldn't. Seeing the film we made of her in June of 2007 made me realise how much I had forgotten, like how she used constantly to blow out through her lips, making a noise that annoyed me and which I used to try to talk to her about, wanting her to stop. I had forgotten so much about that time, trying to erase it, the pain of it, and seeing the film was like seeing myself as a former being. Both of us have changed.

There's a play I once saw, when there were good plays on television, about a vicar in Northern Ireland, an endearing play where he loses his wife, and his daughter is now the only woman in his life, but she is busy with her own family, tending to him and acting as the foil to him for dramatic purposes. Everyone gives him advice on how to pick up his life, which he listens to but he knows he has lost his life's love and does not know why he will carry on. Then one day he is out sweeping up leaves, it is autumn. And as the leaves swirl over his – their – large grounds, he realises that she still speaks to him, that she is the constant in his life, that her spirit is all around and that she never truly went away. He sits there in the autumnal golden light and they play Schubert's First Impromptu in G minor. I am listening to it now and it makes me cry whenever I hear it but for me there is no resolution, not yet. The piece cannot work magic but it always reminds me of widowhood and the possibility of coming to terms with it.

I sit here in a widow's cottage, now a National Trust property let out to people like me, built in 1843 to house the widows and children of men lost at sea. There must have been many tears here, and some relief, to be snug in a cottage built by public subscription. The inner lough empties and fills with a constant rhythm, great flocks of Brent geese and redshank flying to newly exposed sand or to the small island as it is covered or uncovered by the tide. The last time we stayed near water was on Harris, a disastrous holiday, with Irene wanting to paint all the time, which was fine. We had stayed in a bed and breakfast and she had tried to help the landlady make the beds and insisted on asking her for something, I can't remember what – help with mending something? Which at the time I was embarrassed about and tried to dissuade her. I'd already told the landlady about Irene's dementia – her behaviour was so bizarre by then, I had to.

Nothing I read can convey the full magnitude of Alzheimer's – it always seems like an abridged version, losing the full complexity, the confusion, the raw emotion. But Lisa Genova's book *Still Alice* is rightly acclaimed as a good novel. Alice says that for John, her husband, work is his passion in life. She is jolted by this as although they love each other they have these middle-class academic lives where they have each got their own careers and he prioritizes his, as she would have done if she had been well. He is devastated by her diagnosis. For me, Irene was the passion of my life, and work fitted in around it. Sure I made the decision that I could not give up my job; it would make me go mad to be caring at home alone and anyway what would we live on? I would have been around 50, that's all; am only coming up to 55 now, the year we said I would retire and we would go round the world…

Alice gives a speech to the Dementia Care Conference, a wonderfully poignant speech where she explains how it is to be a brilliant academic who is losing her mind. Yet she is left with the essence of her – Still Alice – a person who recognises only love and affection and the true feelings going on around her, not the names of her family or even that they are family. Her plans to commit suicide go by the by, as once you reach that stage you cannot carry it out; you forget what to do.

The whole action takes place over two years, from her starting to realise something is wrong to her becoming unknown to herself, not knowing her husband and kids. This seems too hasty – but not so far different from our experience. Irene was diagnosed in April 2004 but could have been diagnosed two years before that, and hospitalized in August 2007. Milestones, like when Irene said in our kitchen, can you help me with this change? I can't do money any more. She was not perturbed by this, just a statement of fact, as if she was cheerfully handing over a task like counting out the money after a meal with friends in a restaurant, except this was forever, saying she wasn't going to do money any more. She had given £5 for a dozen eggs not expecting any change at the farm. Or not understanding what her watch said, an analogue watch so Gordon bought her a digital one, but that was already too late, and time began not to matter either, like the date. I bought the only clock I could find with the date on it too, a huge thing, but she had already lost the months in her head. When was that? I cannot remember. Yes, I remember the watch – it was for her sixtieth birthday. She has only just turned 62 but it feels like a very long time ago.

It seems strange that we can send probes to Mars, we can scan the minutiae of people's brains, but we cannot understand how anyone else's mind works. Following Irene's mind would be harder than finding our way out of a black hole in another galaxy.

A Further Stage of Dementia

8 February 2010   Irene has taken a dip – well, that's a benign way of describing it. A further stage of dementia, Linda the unit manager said today. It's a euphemism – she clearly thinks it's the end stage. Irene herself doesn't seem distressed, thank God, because if she was I would be distraught. She is not in pain. She cannot seem to open her jaws to eat. She is taking liquids and a small amount of food. I wonder how long this stage lasts? I wonder if she will be here for my 56th birthday. I think not.

She has lost six kilos this month.

I don't know what I feel except sad and upset. I need to weep and I will, but later, alone.

The other day was one of those bizarre days that, if I wasn't so sensitive to the use of words, I would call a demented day. I got to your care home having arranged to meet Jan again for some more filming. I want to capture you again, not for any reason other than it feels right. I was waiting for Jan, and saw a guy in full Scottish traditional dress loitering. Funny how nothing seems out of place there, and I thought nothing except to register 'guy in kilt with bagpipes'. Jan arrived, not feeling well and the day seemed doomed, not because of that but because of some vibe in the air. We went up to find Irene fast asleep on the sofa in the main lounge, and I knew she would not be roused. With Jan, we set about rearranging her room a little to make filming easier, pushing the bed against the wall. I went off to see if Irene had made a miraculous awakening only to have Jino, the in-charge, stop me with a form: 'We still need to look at these end of life papers,' he announced. I was caught between anxious Jan and sleeping Irene and needy Jino, but stopped anyway to explain that I didn't want Irene taken to hospital but for her to stay in her home if she was ill, and if she needed resuscitation not to. Jino went off to write this down and emerged a few minutes later for me to sign. I was making decisions on the hoof, though really it only tidied up what we had been thinking about. Only later did I wonder if they were so concerned about Irene that they wanted the paperwork brought up to date.

Jan came with me with her hand-held camera and I sat trying to work out what was going on with Irene whilst aware of Jan at work, sometimes a lens just inches from my nose or over my shoulder. She wasn't insensitive and we had gone there to film. I felt responsible for her giving up her time but I was also becoming increasingly concerned that Irene wasn't right. She'd had a fit a few days before.

One of the more cantankerous residents, Kath, was poking a small table into the feet of Lyn, who has Down's Syndrome and dementia. Kath kept shouting, 'You can't eat all those bananas', but Lyn didn't budge. Meanwhile, it was dawning on me that Irene was certainly unwell, the cogs in my head whirring, wondering what this might be – the next stage or an infection? What? Then the bagpipes started up, so loud I might have been standing next to the piper. Burns Night of course, and a man in full Scottish regalia is walking through the wing playing to his heart's content. I wonder what the residents made of it. Irene comatose, an unhappy film maker, end of life, no resuscitation, bagpipes, you can't eat all those bananas, Irene being filmed (should she have been?). Everyone would have said such a bizarre run of events could not possibly have been condensed into half an hour.

Then, realising we were not going to get any footage of Irene the person, we retreated to her room and did some filming of me on Irene's bed, Jan asking me questions, the wrong questions, then me walking along her corridor, coming in and out of her room. The film is too late. And it seems silly anyway, in the scale of things. We will have to make do with the footage we already have, and the memories. Irene's life is now beyond us, she has retreated further away.

Today confirmation from the expert, Linda. If Irene doesn't eat, she might only have three weeks to live.

Hard to imagine Irene no longer here, hard to imagine her death, though I have thought of it many times, especially the funeral. She might carry on for some months but I think she won't. She has suddenly slipped away. She looks so tired, a tiredness that has been coming on for a few months, like another falling through thin ice. She has retreated so far.

This week Jean, perhaps her most constant and closest friend, has talked more about her sadness, the loss of her friend. Pauline and Gordon are also concerned. Things are closing in, the final chapter approaches. And me? I ache. My heart aches and I want to cry. The end game, the final stages. A life that could have been so different. A life spent still walking or dining or going to the theatre. Even if for some reason she and I had parted, she might have still been getting those walker's legs up the Lakeland Fells, still musing on a play she'd seen, raving about politics, so many things. Enjoying green-freckled days in the sunshine or rain. Instead she is there on a sofa in track suit bottoms that fall up to her knees as she curls her legs in the air, her mouth gaping open as she sleeps in a lounge with lots of elderly folk, and some only a little older than her, whose lives have also been cruelly shortened, their brains fried and scrambled. The best place for her to be, the most awful place for her to be.

The fit has thrown her off, maybe a cause or a symptom of this latest catastrophic decline. She has not got over it. I want to say, 'Goodnight, sweet girl'.

I have found someone to do Irene's funeral, a humanist and a feminist. I got a list from the Humanist Society. She came out to meet Irene, so she has some sense of her, and Irene, bless her, was on good form that day, her personality was there.

A Further Stage of My Life

In May 2009 I'd summoned up the emotional energy to finish the walk to Land's End, at least the southern part, 104 miles of Cornish landscapes, arriving at Land's End and propping Irene's photo next to my bed in the splendid hotel to which I'd treated myself. I started as the unhappy half of a couple and by the end I realised I'd walked myself into some kind of reasonably contented singledom, with the new-found ease that walking helps to induce. On my return I surprised myself by falling in love with someone and, also to my surprise, she declared, a few weeks later, that she loved me. Not to keep you in suspense, it didn't work out. Our optimism that this meant not having to look for anyone else with whom to share our twilight years with was unfounded. I thought later, as she accompanied me on the final bit of the John o'Groats walking epic, that there was a symbolism, her finishing with me the walk that Irene and I had started so many years before.

Our honeymoon period of nights at the opera and discovering each other's stories didn't materialise into a deeper love. It was she who called it off, in the spring of 2012, and my main feelings were of relief to be out of an emotional tumble dryer. The same trait I have of not giving up even when things were going wrong, which sustained me through looking after Irene, didn't help here. It gave me some happy times though, made me feel alive again, made me look at myself, made me dress up for someone, made me feel wanted by someone. When it ended, it also made me feel like I'd not only rejoined but also joined the human race. I'd had a relationship that had failed, and so I signed up at least to that part of the human race that scours the room for an ex at a social gathering and who leaves friends in a dilemma about which one of us to invite. And for more than two years, I had constant confused dreams about Irene being out of the care home, ill but somehow out on licence, and I didn't know what she understood, but I knew that I would have to explain that I was seeing someone else now, and she would have to go back to the care home. But in those years, I also had a girlfriend, someone who helped me through some hard times with Irene, and who would also visit Irene with me. We went through two fractured ankles and the major scare of Irene's illness in the late winter of 2010, when we thought Irene was going to die. And she did not die. She confounded everyone by pulling through that illness when she looked like death warmed up, as we used to say as children.

Those years saw progressive losses. From being such a walker, Irene's legs went in the early summer of 2011. In fine weather, I would always take Irene outside into the lovely grounds and we would walk, or sit in the sunshine. In the autumn, I would pick blackberries there as she would stand by. She started to falter, her eyes not seeing how to cross lines or step off kerbs. The home is large, with three parts, the Memory Lane Community, the frail elderly unit and a wing for people with physical disabilities, MS, spinal injuries and so on. We would walk through it all, getting to know all sorts of residents and staff. Irene was always on the move, though I could also coax her to stop and sit on a private sofa somewhere, or on a bench outside and we could have time to ourselves. Losing the ability to walk meant suddenly this stopped, giving a different shape and feel to my visits. Walking was the centre of our shared life together before Irene was ill, and it carried on after she went into care that we would walk, even if only up and down, so it was hard when it stopped. She seemed happy enough though. Harder still for me was when the staff started to put Irene into a big comfy wheelchair, in the spring of 2012, with a strap to stop her falling out. I hated this latest act of confinement. But it did mean I could wheel her outside, giving us the chance to sit in the sunshine again.

Walking gone. Words too. I wrote a poem back in 2008:

You Were an English Teacher

You were an English teacher,
Knew about onomatopoeia, alliteration,
Could write in iambic pentameter,
Count the syllables for a haiku in your head.

'What day is it?' 'Monday.'
Words came easily,
All the remembered conversations.

'What day is it?' 'Monday.'
You wrote funny letters and made up rhymes,
Could be relied on for a leaving speech,
Taught me how to do the Guardian cryptic crossword.
'What day is it?' 'Monday.'

Gone from your head, the names and words.
'What day is it?'
'Still Monday.'
For this there are no words.

Now words have really gone. At least, intelligible words. Any dialogue ceased almost as soon as Irene went into care, but at least she said things to us, and I, we, said things to her. It's a long time since Irene said the words I liked to hear, though she would sometimes look at me and just say, 'I…' and I knew what she meant to say to me. It was OK; I know she still loves me, without the words. Words were such a big part of Irene's life – she loved them, thought about them, exuberated in them. Some people at the home still have normal speech; you can have a conversation, even if it's forgotten 30 seconds later. So strange, this disease. When Irene speaks, so softly, murmuring her own 'words', it's so poignant it makes me want to cry. Her little voice. Once you could have heard Irene at the other end of a school hall.

The other thing that has fallen off is people visiting Irene. Now there's only me, her brother, her good old university friend and two friends she used to work with. It has hurt that so many of our friends' visits declined many years ago. I can understand that it's distressing to see Irene now and easier to remember her as she was, but. I've talked about it with my confidantes. They say it is hard and it's not surprising that people don't feel able to visit. Some people don't see the point if Irene 'doesn't recognize them' or that she wouldn't know they'd been anyway. Others just feel inadequate, scared, unsure what to do. And I want to say: just hold her hand. Just sit with her and she might know that there is someone there who cares about her, that for she who lives in the omnipresent present, no future and no past, every minute where an extra ounce of happiness might be squeezed out is a bonus. But I don't. I swallow my hurt and just organize little tea parties from time to time so that people can see her in the safety of a small group. I don't want anyone to be left with the regret of knowing that they turned out for her funeral but didn't bother to see her when she was still alive.

Others, less part of an inner circle (and even those in it) do ask after her. They say, 'Oh well, remember me to her – would she remember me?' And I mumble something to the effect that she often doesn't know who I am. They look at me, saddened. No one can have any idea unless they see it for themselves.

I made the trip to New Zealand to see Arafelle, spending a week on her smallholding. Her partner had died before I went, and she had a terrible story to tell of family dispossession, of hours to drive to see her lovely partner in care, of not being told when she had died in 2008. We talked and talked, though I was also strangely muted about Irene, not yet able to find the words.

So, my new beginning turned out to be a cul-de-sac, or maybe a side road. It was wonderful to find someone to love and be loved and, although it didn't last, it brought me back to the main road a little higher up, further along the way, and a happier person. I never left Irene during those years. I saw her as much, cared for her as much, but somehow being single again and without distractions brought me back to her in a profound way. I saw her more clearly than I had for a while and was acutely aware again of what we'd had. The grief, never far away, socked me in the jaw with all its might. It may be a conceit to claim this as a 'special relationship' – after all, many have such a thing. But I do know that what we had wasn't ordinary; losing a super-ordinary love leads to super-ordinary loss and to super-ordinary grief. No wonder it has such enduring power.

I read that when the love of Tennessee Williams' life, his long-term partner Frank Merlo, died in the early 1960s, Williams never really recovered, though he lived another 20 years. They adored each other. I'm not sure why I find this comforting, but I do. I also know that once you've had one great love there's no reason why you shouldn't have another, and that's what you'd want for me, and what I'd want for you, were our roles reversed.. Someone to wake up beside and say 'Hey gorgeous'. Not a lot to ask, is it?

Amy Loid and Her Cronies

It's 2012, and I have developed a little more hardiness about understanding this disease that you have, my poor love. Time to face the barrage of amyloids.

I read that Alzheimer's disease is characterized by a dramatic loss of neurons and synapses, especially in the hippocampus and cortex. There is a poetry of science and I haven't really a clue what this means, but I'm glad someone does. It seems that the disease causes a mutation in three genes: amyloid-β protein precursor (AβPP), presenilin-1, and presenilin-2. These genetic changes result in fragments depositing themselves as plaques, and this is what causes the damage. I like the word 'amyloid' and especially an amyloid cascade. Irene and I would weave this into a story that could run for days: Amy Loid and her coterie, cascading – no, parachuting – into people's lives like a cheeky, wicked gremlin, causing 'missense mutations', creating abnormalities and extracellular accumulation, like extracurricular activities leading to blissful perversities. Well, maybe not.

And the scientific papers talk of familial and sporadic origins. Was Irene's disease sporadic or familial? We will never know. Her mother had an unusual horror of dementia. She herself was slightly more than normally forgetful in later life, and would write things carefully down on her calendar, both things that had happened and were about to happen, knowing that she could not trust her memory. She was mortified when the husband of one of her best friend's developed dementia. He could no longer remember the rules of the card games they played and everyone turned away, wounded, embarrassed, sorrowful. Irene's father had all his marbles until his death from a stroke. Her mother had died 11 months previously, doing the classic dropping dead of a heart attack on her way back from posting a letter on a too-cold December day. But her genetic origins are shadowy and forever unknowable, the child of a First World War liaison between a working class girl in Manchester and an officer. When this child, Joyce, Irene's mother, was three, she was given away to an unpleasant, Victorian sort of woman in the neighbourhood. Joyce was old enough to understand; she tried to walk back to her previous home, where her birth mother had taken up with a man who did not want reminders of his new wife's past. Later, Joyce nursed an anger that did not leave her in old age, the fury in her eyes about 'that woman', her birth mother. Her adopted parents (though I doubt the arrangement was ever formalised) were harsh and I believe she was treated like a skivvy. Her redemption was finding work in a shop once her education was terminated, and in the Manchester Ramblers' Club, where so many working class people from the back streets of Manchester and other northern towns found freedom and fun on their one day off at the weekend. There she met Jack, a fine walker from a more respectable background than she. They married and when Irene was four and her older brother seven, they realised their dream of leaving Manchester and finding jobs in the Lake District, Jack as a chemical analyst with the Freshwater Biological Institute. His job was to analyse the waters of the lakes and tarns, and from four years old Irene was hiked up and down the Lakeland fells, beginning a love affair with that part of the world, and with walking, that endured. When she was striding ahead and I struggled to keep up, I would joke that she was bred for walking – there was no wonder I could only straggle behind. Apart from that, I know nothing of her breeding, of her genetic makeup.

Maybe it's not genetic anyway, but the sporadic type. Sporadic – it means erratic, random, irregular, periodic. There will never be a reason, never be a satisfactory answer to the 'Why her?' question. There never is and, anyway, 'shit happens' says the T-shirt. Jacqueline du Pré got Multiple Sclerosis didn't she? Where's the fairness in that? None. Just got to get on with it.

Whatever the reason, Irene's brain was set upon by Amy Loid and her cronies, peptide and stuff, leading to neuropathological alterations which defeated both of us. We could not outpace the aberrant accumulation, though we had a good stab at slowing it down, with the Aricept and our ruthless determination to carry on with life as normal. Aricept, or its generic name, donezepil, increases hippocampal volume, whatever that is, and it did work, slowing the speed of Irene's decline. But it's like holding back the tide – it works for a while and then is overcome. However it worked, maybe giving us an extra year or more of quality time. The National Institute for Clinical Excellence (NICE) tried to stop its prescription due to insufficient evidence. Had we been asked, we could have provided some. Irene was put on to Aricept way before NICE made its controversial decision. After the public anger, the Health Secretary of the day, Labour's John Reid, intervened to suggest that NICE needed to look again at the data. In a face-saving move, NICE agreed that maybe there was data that would suggest a different picture and in time the verdict on four dementia drugs was changed. As the press noted at the time, the drugs in question cost about £2.50 per person per day, so around £1,000 per year. I reckon they enabled Irene to remain at home for at least another year, giving us valuable time together. As to the financial benefit, that would have saved around £11,000, giving a net benefit of £10,000. Even if it was true that Aricept only worked in half the cases, the savings are impressive and for that 50-60 per cent of sufferers where benefits accrue, they last for up to 18 months.

However, these drugs need to be given early on and what seems to happen in the UK is that getting to a diagnosis takes longer than in other European countries. In Germany, for example, the average time is 10 months while in Britain it's 32. In the UK, only 20 per cent of people with Alzheimer's are offered drugs – in Italy it's 80 per cent. Why such differences? These drugs, Aricept, Exelon, Reminyl, all seem to be useful in the mild to moderate stages, and Ebixa in the moderate to severe stages.

At first, NICE welcomed these drugs but either it did not have the full picture or it made an error of judgment. Moreover, the accounting tools appeared only to consider a narrow range of measures. Carers' quality of life didn't seem to come into the equation. And how do you measure the fact that a person with dementia can remember their grandchildren's names for another year, or can walk down to the newsagent's on their own to buy a pint of milk?

There's a point where it's right to stop a drug if it's no longer having an effect but what seems controversial is the test to assess this. It didn't happen in Irene's case – her decline when she went into care was so spectacular that she could not have been tested. In most cases, however, the MMSE (mini mental state examination) is applied to assess whether someone is still in the mild to moderate stage and therefore likely to benefit. Patients are asked some pretty difficult questions, such as to count backwards from 100 in sevens, or to remember an address and repeat it a few minutes later. I'm not sure I could easily do that now, in the relaxed comfort of my own home. To do so in a state of anxiety, under scrutiny of a medical team, where I know I'm being set up to fail is obviously harder. Failing means the drugs might be stopped.

The pharmaceutical industry of course has an incentive to see more people take their drugs. And with so much dementia around, they see new developments as a way to refresh their portfolios, as the financial pages report. Experimental compounds are bought for undisclosed sums. A piece in the *Guardian* (13 July 2012) said AstraZeneca had given itself three years to make its new neuroscience division work, with 40 staff 'largely relying on external collaborations and partnerships'. Although the headline is 'AstraZeneca focuses on brain disease treatments', the article went on to say that '900 neuroscientists have been laid off and half the brain disease products in development scrapped to make way for the new virtual approach'. It seems these nimbler units, quality over quantity, is now the way to come up with new drugs in this exceptionally high-risk area.

Risk to profits, that is, not the risk that more and more people will succumb before there's sufficient funding to forge ahead on some real breakthroughs.

Drugs aside, there are occasional titbits in the health sections of newspapers about staving off dementia, meeting a demand from readers for more lifestyle approaches to it. 'What can I do?' people seem be imploring. In the Doctor's Dilemmas page, someone asked 'Should I eat chocolate to relieve dementia?' The reassuring reply was that as so many people have some form of dementia (1 in 14 people over the age of 65, according to the Alzheimer's Society) there are many studies examining how it can be stopped from progressing. That's good then! And, a recent study in the journal Hypertension showed that in a sample of 91 people aged over 70 with mild impairment, some improved on cognitive tests when they were given high and medium concentration cocoa drinks, compared with those given only low concentration cocoa drinks. Seemingly, the cocoa lowers blood pressure and resistance to insulin, which means that the body gets better at absorbing high levels of glucose – which can reduce the progress of dementia. Later in the article: 'The study was funded by Mars, which doesn't mean it was biased, but the company would have preferred to find chocolate has a positive effect'. (*Guardian* 20 August 2012).

More Debates

There are other debates as the rates of dementia increase. It seems a huge injustice that once a person develops dementia they are seen as needing social care, not necessarily health care. In Irene's case we were awarded so-called continuing care, i.e. care needed as a result of a health issue. In other cases, an elderly person is considered not as a health case but as a social one, someone who simply can no longer look after themselves (at least in England and Wales. Scotland took a different route and pays for social care– though there are now questions as to whether it can afford to continue doing so). I sort of knew that I wouldn't lose my house, and that somehow Irene's care would be paid for, but it left a lot of anxiety. It's crazy that I should have to worry about whether her care would be paid for when she was struck down by a vile disease that happened to be a dementia. It would not have been a worry at all had it been a brain tumour or motor neurone disease.

How to look after people in the later stages of their lives is a matter of huge debate, one I can't go into here and really it's about how we treat our elderly people in general. But Irene wasn't elderly. There was a headline in our local paper about the council turning down a proposal from a developer about using a piece of land to build more care facilities for people with dementia. The council thought that such a move would lead to property prices sliding and would degrade the value of the land. Readers were asked to write in, so I did, lamenting the lack of places for younger people with dementia.

I read an item about a place called Hogewey in Holland. It houses 152 residents with severe or extreme dementia. Finished in 2010, it's described as:

A compact, self-contained model village on a four-acre site on the outskirts of town, half of it open space: wide boulevards, cosy side-streets, squares,

143

sheltered courtyards, well-tended gardens with ponds, reeds and a profusion of wild flowers. The rest is neat, two-storey, brick-built houses, as well as cafe, restaurant, theatre, minimarket and hairdressing salon.

People live in 23 homes, each decorated to suit the resident, and each with their own room and bathroom and a shared kitchen, lounge and dining room. It's staffed by 250 full- or part-time staff. There's lots to do and people are free to wander. There are no locked areas, no keypads and no security codes. Residents can ride bikes, be out in the sunshine, play boules, buy an ice cream – in short, do all the normal things they would be doing if they were still at home and not ill, except that they are safe and looked after. The home has 25 clubs centred on anything from folk music to baking, and residents join in ordinary activities, like folding the laundry, gardening – things they have always done and which require only muscle memory.

The whole thing doesn't cost any more to run than a conventional care home and people living there use less medication. One of those behind it commented: 'I think maybe we've shown that even if it is cheaper to build the kind of care home neither you nor I would ever want to live in, the kind of place where we've looked after people with dementia for the last 30 years or more, we perhaps shouldn't be doing it anymore.' (*Guardian* 28 August 2012)

I've always been happy with Irene's care home. I sing its praises and the staff are terrific. I can get emotional when I think of them, day after day, doing their job with such cheerfulness, respect, kindness and skill. There are little touches, such as always having a printed menu card on each table in the dining room even though most of the residents cannot read it. The food is great and there's plenty of it. The rooms are like hotel rooms really. The furnishings are not worn; the place is spruce, colourful. That criterion that's so often invoked – 'Does it smell of urine?' – isn't an issue. Outside there's an enclosed courtyard and around the building are gardens and trees. There are lots of events – Halloween, Easter, harvest, summer fayres and so on – and entertainers come in regularly. I've had some wonderful times there at social events and it's a place where everyone is accepted for just exactly who and what they are. Of its kind, it's an excellent place and I'd recommend it. Of its kind. Hmm…

Would I want to end up there?

Reading about Hogewey, I realise that if all we're ever offered is apples, even excellent apples, we won't know there are oranges. And that there is a different way of looking after people with dementia.

I can see now, reading about Hogewey, that Irene's care home is on the traditional model, a large living area where residents do indeed sit a lot of the time; a dining room; small lounges too; and bedrooms off the main corridors. The Memory Lane Community is a locked one and there are people who would be perfectly able to go outside if they were allowed to do so and if that 'outside' was enclosed. Instead they have to make do with a balcony or be taken out by a staff member, and sadly those staff can't afford to do much one-to-one escorting, so people tend to stay indoors. However much the staff has tried to make it a home, it remains an institution.

I read that people are flocking to Weesp, half an hour south-east of Amsterdam, to see it for themselves. I might go myself.

I can't help wondering how much of Irene's steep decline after she was admitted to the acute psychiatric hospital was because of the conditions of that place. With its dark corridors and bedrooms (more like cells) off them, its bare walls, it felt like some kind of penal institution. She knew, the morning after, that she was being sent away as she kept saying she had done nothing wrong – she thought she was being put in prison. So she had awareness at that point. If she had gone to a Hogewey instead, what might have been the result?

Madness lies in asking too many 'what-ifs' but madness also lies in carrying on as we are. Already we spend more than £23 billion each year caring for people with dementia; already a quarter of UK hospital beds are occupied by people with dementia; and already we spend three times as much on dementia as on heart disease. Isn't it worth asking the questions and seeing if we could do it differently?

And isn't there a better way of caring for people in those crazy stages of dementia before they need institutional care? Looking back, I realise the dangers and the difficulties of that time for me and Irene. Some problems need only a bucket of hot soapy water, as when Irene was confused one night and crouched by my side of the bed, peeing on the carpet. Others could have ended in disaster, like the time in Norfolk when she took off on her bike: by the time I'd realised she wasn't coming back, she'd gained on me and it took me an hour to catch her up, on a busy A-road. I saw her ahead of me and she didn't have a clue where she was or where she was going. Another time in Scotland, she leapt from the car and by the time I'd parked, I'd lost her. I saw her on a street below after more than a half-hour of frantic searching. She was getting into a car with a man. I ran behind the car madly waving and he stopped. He was going to take her to the police station, a Good Samaritan, not some maniac rapist as it turned out. The husband of my friend in the village, 80 and with Alzheimer's, left the house in the middle of the night recently and was brought back by the police. She now has to lock the bedroom door.

These are ordinary incidents and we are left to deal with them. If the figures are to be believed (which presumably they can, as they come from Oxford University and would they tell porkies?), we will have one million people with dementia by 2025. That means a similarly large number of people caring for them at home in those years leading up to the need for care. The toll on those partners, daughters, sons will be immense, leading to the sort of health problems that Joan developed.

I don't know what the answers are – some element of risk necessarily goes with the territory. If you are trying to keep someone at home, or if they don't need care yet, there will be times when something potentially disastrous happens. Yet what we have is carers who are largely unsupported, untrained, floundering, and with total responsibility for the welfare of not only another human being but one who holds their heart strings. A human being who behaves outside the normal rules of conduct, who becomes a law unto themselves and who does things you have no idea how to deal with, except to fall back on your wits. It's often when the carers can no longer cope, or the care they have put in place falls apart, that the demented person gets more attention from the statutory services. It doesn't resonate well with person-centred care.

A Media Deluge

When I spoke to a confidante about whether anyone would ever read my book, she said, 'Well there's so much about Alzheimer's, it's in the media every day, it pops up all the time'. Indeed, when I open my email at the moment, a message comes unbidden on the page, in the annoying right hand column of adverts, 'Spot the early signs of dementia. Keep the person you know and love a little bit longer'. It's next to a photo of a smiling older woman. The logic of the two sentences appears to need no further elaboration. How does knowing the early signs lead to keeping them longer? The early signs aren't much different from what a lot of middle-aged women go through in the menopause – a series of small but significant changes, a faltering, a bit of depression. Hard to spot and even harder to diagnose. Maybe nothing, maybe normal, maybe potentially devastating.

Dementia is indeed in the media a lot. The news from the drugs industry that hits the papers from time to time creates a surge of hope in my science fiction-indulged brain that a miracle cure will come and Irene will somehow be restored. Even the most phantasmagorical element in me knows this is completely improbable. It feels that little leprechaun that wants to pop out and say, 'Ha, fooled you! We were only joking, she's fine really'. And it also makes me feel sad that, for Irene, everything is too late.

The other way dementia hits the newspapers is in stories of all the others for whom it's too late, about those caring for someone with dementia, about someone famous with it or, very occasionally, by someone who has it themselves. There's always a common story, elements that resonate with all of us in the dementia community. So it's good these stories are told – they let us know that we're in this together.

Stuart Jeffery (*Guardian* 1 April 2006) wrote a beautiful testimony to his mother, who developed dementia in her nineties. He talks of how they measured their visits to her, '"not too bad today", which meant she might have said one word in an hour of mumbles, this being 'one more word than the week before'. He notes how she could be unintentionally funny in her speech, but how 'her unusual responses achieved more than normal speech'. I know what he means – sometimes in Irene's stumbling words she would say something which was so profound. Yet it would have sounded trite or cheesy if she'd meant it, like when she said 'I am you and you are me'. Jeffery's mother once said: 'I must be losing my bonkers!' and 'A man came in with a very important moustache'. He advises writing as much down as possible and the reason he could write the article was because he's an inveterate scribbler. He advises: 'Note down what you can while speech lasts, because it can tide you over while you wait for the glass of the past to clear and for memories of how people were to come flooding back. At least, that is my hope.' I know I could not have held on to all this unless I had written it down; at the time it was just a release. Now it's a record, a way of holding on. Losing your mum or dad as part of the cycle of life and death is awful. Losing them to dementia is heartbreaking. But losing a parent is what is supposed to happen – they are meant to die before us. It's normal. I know I can do normal grief because that's what happened when my own mum died in 2004. She had been ill with all sorts, she was in full possession of her faculties – but her body had given out. She was ready to go. I will always miss her but my grief has run its course, did so long ago. Latterly we'd had a good relationship, leaving me with no regrets, no unfinished business. So I know I can do normal. My grief for Irene is different and when people know about our story and say, 'Oh yes, I know how you feel, my mum/dad had dementia', I smile sympathetically but inside I want to throttle them. Losing a partner, and losing one to early onset, is not the same.

At the other extreme from Stuart Jeffery's mother, there's a story about Mark Priddy. 'It was 2005, and Mark, aged 36, had just been diagnosed with early onset Alzheimer's. Less than a year later, he was moved into a care home, where he became unable to walk, talk or feed himself. Five years later, he died.' (*Guardian* 6 October 2012) The story centres on his wife Dione, and their two daughters, who were only primary school age. Thirty-six! That's the youngest I've heard of, and inevitably the article produces a statistic – 15,000 people under 65 with dementia in the UK.

There is the usual pattern of funny behaviour, like putting the knives and forks in the bin instead of washing them up, and this family does seem to have had as much fun as they could squeeze out in the time left. They renewed their marriage vows, which Mark seemed to value, but that evening Mark asked Dione, 'Are you a nurse?' Dione berates herself for not telling the children sooner, that old question of who and what to tell. As with us, she says that when she and Mark were told, she couldn't take it in that he had dementia. She doesn't say whether she discussed it with him.

Mark was first prescribed anti-depressants, as was Irene. How many GPs, seeing such early onset, will think about Alzheimer's? Even if it's supposedly common, they might see one or two cases on their patch in their whole career. Eventually Mark was sectioned; he had 'mood swings, terrifying them all with temper tantrums'. Though the phrase 'temper tantrums' somehow infantilises, it is a good description – people with Alzheimer's can do spectacular tantrums and sadly it's one of the main things friends and I remember and talk about. ('Do you remember the time in that ice cream shop when Irene …') I know that with Irene there were happy times, times of relative calm, such as painting peacefully, but what's wearing about being with someone in that phase is that you never know what's going to happen next, so you're in a state of nervous anticipation all the time.

Erasing the dramas and the traumas is tough, and letting memories flood back of the good times, the time before the illness (which goes on for so long!) is a struggle. So, from a mum in her nineties to a husband in his thirties. Extremes certainly, but some common threads in that first puzzlement, that inability to quite put your finger on what's wrong. Then a diagnosis, shock, and a stunning fall if you're younger and a slower more imperceptible decline if you're older.

And the famous people? How great it is when they feel they can go public – something that so many don't feel able to do, as if it's something to be ashamed of. That's why what Terry Pratchett did, brave, brave man, is so amazing. Irene once stunned us, at a gathering of Labour Party friends, when everyone knew she had Alzheimer's (so maybe 2005), by saying, 'Isn't it sad about Margaret Thatcher having Alzheimer's?' There was silence in the room for a few seconds before anyone knew how to respond. How she knew that I don't know – it was years before anything was said about the Iron Lady and way before the film let it all out.

Secrets are best let out. There's a coming-out story which incidentally throws up a dementia story. The first (in 2012!), brave (there are homophobic murders there, including that of a close friend) openly gay boxer, Orlando

Cruz, from Puerto Rico recalls Emile Griffith 50 years previously, who was also gay but could not come out. Later Griffith developed dementia. In 1962 he was taunted by an opponent, Benny Paret, as a 'faggot' and Griffith pounded him so badly in the fight that Paret died 10 days later. Griffith observed: 'I kill a man and most people forgive me. I love a man and most people say this makes me an evil person'.

Glen Campbell's farewell tour is a brave act. A journalist wrote:

> *As we chat, Campbell sits contentedly singing to himself, half listening. I ask him if*
> *he is worried about touring because of the Alzheimer's.*
> *'Where did that come up? That Alzheimer?' he says.*
> *'You were diagnosed with Alzheimer's,' Kim [his wife] says gently.*
> *Campbell: 'Oh, I was? Well. No, no I don't worry.'*

And he doesn't need to worry, as he has the songs and the music in his head, laid down in some part of his brain that is still intact. His wife says touring fills his life with meaning.

Irene is Lasting

2012   The cast has been changing. It's imperceptible when you judge it week by week but, when you look back over months, you realise that some faces are no longer there. There's Roy who, when he first arrived, would sing with gusto, a lovely baritone in the middle of the main lounge. Now he's bedridden and sometimes, his door open so that he can have some sense of comings and goings, his stick-like legs protrude from under the duvet. More than half the original cast I wrote about earlier has died. Another Margaret is there and she has the voice of an aristocrat, imperiously shouting out commands, as if to a chauffeur. She is tiny, immobile, and her beady eyes don't miss a thing. She once was sitting opposite me and Irene, and she was scolding me but out of concern for Irene. She said, 'Can't you do something about her, can't you see she's ill? You need to take her home!' and so on. It was a time after Irene stopped walking and the staff would willingly have moved either her or Irene but I just sat it out. There's Fraser who collects things, places them on a sofa and sits amidst them all. He's a large man and it's difficult to prise objects back from him; the shortage of spoons in the dining room is all due to him. The staff never tell me, unless I ask, if someone has died. Instead I get all the gossip from Angela, a year older than Irene who, when asked, says she's 24 and has a fiancé called Michael. She is articulate and somehow unlike the others; she seems to have had learning disabilities all her life but she always knows who I am. She also knows what goes on, and will suddenly blurt out, 'X has died' or 'X has had a stroke', or 'Ooh, that noisy old sod, he fell down the other day'.

No one seems to have told these folk what their average life expectancy with dementia was meant to be. Some are there for years and years in a state where you think they cannot possibly survive much longer.

Some come in and go quickly, still, it would seem, fit and otherwise healthy. And that psychiatrist's statement, delivered so long ago, meant, I suppose, as a kindly thought, that 'People with Alzheimer's live an average of eight or nine years', is often at the back of my mind. At the time I was stunned. Later I wanted to say 'but how can you possibly produce such a statistic – it's meaningless!' First, the diagnosis might come only months or it could be years into the illness, so when do you start counting those years that are left? Also the sloppy use of 'average' – mean, median or mode? 'Come on man, what exactly do you mean?' I should have barked. A mean is just a piece of arithmetic. Those with dementia just do their thing, keep going despite the odds, or give up, or just plain die of something else.

The staff too has changed, though not greatly – turnover is small, which I take as a good sign. The staff forms the proverbial microcosm of modern English life. The care assistants are strong Polish men with tattoos who wear those chunky silver bracelets and smoke, who you would worry about meeting in a dark alley but who care for their charges with such tenderness, like watching a bear gently moving her cubs. There are young Yorkshire lasses who chat among themselves about dieting, whose mums would probably never take any nonsense from them and who treat their charges with the respect they would give a much loved gran or granddad. There are young Filipino women, all with dark hair, all with a delicacy of touch. One has painted the stairs up to the Memory Lane Community with a profusion of tropical flowers and grasses, invoking her knowledge of a home she will one day return to.

The more senior staff on the unit with team leadership roles are working class from around about. They are irrepressibly cheerful, down-to-earth; nothing fazes them. Wrong to single any out, but here are two: the amazing Jan who tells me she likes my hair, or who says I look well, who sings and is a bundle of energy; and Wayne, marvellously camp, does terrific Diana Ross impersonations at the many dances and has kindness printed, like Blackpool rock, through his tall thin body. The qualified in-charges, those who do the drugs rounds and who tell me what's happening for Irene, are either English, Indian or from southern Africa. These are the staff who phone me after Irene has had another fit, which she has more and more of, and who tell me about changing Irene's various dosages. These are the staff who sit in on the yearly review meetings with social services and the ones who now know Irene better than I do. They are all serene, sensitive, efficient. No wonder Irene relaxed as soon as she arrived in this place, took to it immediately.

There's a different feel from the previous, hectic, community unit with its care-worn and over-worked staff.

Then there's the hospitality staff, the ones who make the place run like a hotel, and the reception staff, the cleaners, and the laundry staff, and the two handymen and drivers. After four and a half years, they all recognize me if I bump into them in the supermarket. Some I have got to know well and it will be strange not to see them once I no longer need to visit. And the manager's welcome smile I will always appreciate and cherish. She has now got the OLGA logo on the back of the company's leaflets, a battle she took on and won. OLGA – Older Lesbian and Gay Association.

The staff experiment with the rooms and there have been various refits over the years. Fairly recently, Irene was in the sensory room. It had a projection on the wall, porthole-shaped, of various dolphins and fish that loomed up in a moving sequence, fluorescent straw-thin light showers and mood music. If Irene had been at all conscious, she'd have been very confused about where she was meant to be (am I at sea?) but as she was, I don't think she was aware at all...So it might have been better to have sat her near the kitchens and maybe those smells (smell seems to be the most emotive of all our senses) of baking and bacon might have provided more comfort, and at no cost.

Now I nearly always coincide my visits with meal times. It helps to have a task to do. Often Irene doesn't know anyone is there. She seems so, so tired.

Some posters have been put up on the stairs up to Irene's floor. They are from the Alzheimer's Society. There's one of stones in a river which says, 'Everybody is different but we all have much in common'. Another shows an elderly lady with her arms outstretched over a large bubble, as if to catch it, with the words, 'We spend life as a human being not as a human doing'. And: 'Become like a butterfly – change the moment' with a picture of a large butterfly. 'Accept someone as they are – embrace their reality', with a woman gazing at a doll. 'Reflect on your congruence in being person-centred', with a picture of the back of a man's head. 'Realise it is all about your feelings from now on', with a woman touching some flowers. I read them each time I walk up those stairs, must be dozens of times now, and each time I wonder if some of them, will, one day, suddenly make even the teeniest bit of sense. Or maybe they too are meant to be ever so slightly demented.

Two incidents: I bumped into someone I hadn't seen for ages at a Hugh Masekela concert. I was telling her that I had been seeing someone but that it had ended and my main feeling was of relief. She concurred and said, 'Yes, I can see why, she was very demanding.' I said, 'Oh, I didn't think you had met her,' and she said, 'Yes I did, I met her several times'. I realised she was talking about Irene, not my girlfriend. She knew Irene's diagnosis. I told my chum Laura and she hugged me and said, 'Oh no! She has no idea about loyalty and long relationships!' Quite.

The milk lady who has known us for 25 years asked how Irene was. I told her (though I never know quite what to say, and usually just make something up) and she asked how often I see her. I said every four or five days. She looked shocked, 'Wow, that's a lot, four or five days?' 'Yes,' said I. 'Well,' she said, 'we used to see someone up there about once a month.' Yes, I thought, teeth clenching and wanting to say, 'She's my partner, she's not "someone" and what's more if that was your husband, you would see him every few days.'... But I couldn't say any of that or I would have burst into tears. 'She's been in there five years now,' I said instead.

I found something I wrote in 2008. Would I still stand by it in 2012? Yes, of course:

'If we knew what was round the corner in life – and if we knew that that future contained Alzheimer's – would we despair? Probably, so it's just as well that we don't know the future. I was lamenting to my sister-in-law that I was grieving for our future together, that I wanted another 30 years of our retirement together rather than just our 30 years of life so far, and she said well, you don't know that would have happened anyway – Irene might have died from something else, or canoed off into the sunset with someone else (unlikely, but you never know). I found this surprisingly cheering. What I do know is that even if I had known that we were to be sent the script with Alzheimer's written into the story line instead of the script that I'd hoped for, I would still have chosen to spend my life with Irene, the best partner anyone could ever have wished for.'

20 October 2012   Irene was in bed in her room when I went in yesterday. It was 4.30 in the afternoon and she hadn't been up. They seem to be leaving her in bed now some days. I don't know if the fits she has every few months are weakening her. Other residents don't seem to have them. For several weeks the staff have been talking to me in such a way that tells me they are trying to tell me something. They do this, gently, in a kind of code. They are all doing it now, the nurses in charge. One day they took Irene down to the part of the unit reserved for the really ill people and they explained they thought it might be more peaceful for her. Now they are saying that if she's more comfortable, they leave her in bed. I have to admit that it's reached the point where it's harder to see Irene like this than it is to contemplate her gone. Of the two sets of awfulness, the least awful is for her to be released from this. She would hate it, hate seeing herself like this. Joan, another resident, wandered in lopsidedly while I was giving Irene her meal, reciting, 'Come on, come on,' over and over, trying to get someone to go somewhere with her, as usual. She's looking for her husband, who lives downstairs in the frail elderly unit. They are devoted to each other.

It's crept up on us – Irene being bedridden. I realise with a jolt that it's 18 months since she stopped walking. She looks like a 90 year-old, not a 65 year-old. Her bed is as low to the floor as possible so she doesn't fall out. She suddenly seems so institutionalized, in a nightie I didn't recognize. I have been dreading her being bedridden. She is so thin, gaunt, but she ate well. The staff always say, 'She's eating well.' When I arrived she was quite agitated, and held on to my sweater, pulling it. I don't know if she wanted something – I cannot tell any more. She just lies there, all day, her life reduced to – nothing? But her grip is strong, almost impossible to prise off if she grips my hand, or my collar.

Someone told me that the strength of a person's grip tells you how strong they are, a surrogate measure of how long they might last.

You are lasting. I am lasting.

Our last goodbye is still to come and I've no idea when. I have written what I want to say at the funeral. I have chosen music. I do not want to be caught by surprise. I want it to be good, which means I have to plan now, as at the time I will be a wreck. I am dreading it. Time to 'Stop all the clocks', time for the handkerchiefs, the time when ambiguous loss will turn to certain loss.

31 October 2012 Deia I have written it all out. It's a book, whether it gets published or not. I do feel better, lighter, like when I leave a counselling session, as if some weight has been left behind. It's like looking through the wrong end of my binoculars, everything further away. I can be happy – though only if I don't think of it too much. I'm OK.

But it stuns me, this grief of mine that runs so deeply, still. I would still love to have you back. I can sob just as deeply as ever whenever I think of you and what we've lost, even though you have now been gone from home for five years and you have gone in so many other senses. This grief is a well that never empties. But I get on with life and there are good times; what I seem to know is that happiness and sadness can co-exist, that the joy and wonder of life can mingle with the most dreadful depths of grieving. And I also am beginning to understand that maybe life is all about reconciling ourselves, gracefully, to what we cannot have.

A False Ending!

Alzheimer's has this habit of creating false endings, like a plane coming in to land then suddenly taking off again, and so leaving you up in the air when you thought you'd reached solid ground. That was a false ending to my book too!

On the way home, in the *Sun* newspaper left on a plane seat, there was an article about a poor man with dementia, in his eighties, who killed his beloved nephew with a kitchen knife, as he mistook him for an intruder.

And the Prime Minister is talking about tackling the problem of growing numbers of people with dementia, the need to address the stigma of it – great. But he talks about creating an army of a million volunteers who can help take care of those with dementia, and my heart sinks. Really? Will this do it? Stop people mistaking their nephew for an intruder, occupy Irene for hours, keep her safe? A million volunteers means about one each for everyone who will have dementia.

And I realise that the conclusion to what I wrote in Deia is only a part of the story, that life is always more complicated. How do I simultaneously value what I've been through these last years yet want to wipe it all out by simply having you back? All my struggles and learning, and I'm reminded of a TV series seen long ago called Late Starter, about a man who retired from academia but, inexplicably, his wife deserted him the same day. He learned over the following weeks that she was a compulsive gambler and had systematically gone through every bit of money they'd had. He had to leave his house, get a job as a bartender. His life was thoroughly turned upside down. He was a late starter and actually found a richness that he'd not known before. And when finally, his wife did re-enter his life briefly, he realised actually he preferred the course of events that had happened rather than the one he was expecting. I don't feel like that, but I have found certain riches too, my life having gone on a disquieting new trajectory. It all seems so

157

long ago that I had a normal life with Irene. I have moved on because that is what time does to you. I am immersed in what I have now and the thought of going back to something from a previous life seems a bigger step back than I can visualise. I don't want to mythologise our shared past. But would I prefer to have you in my life rather than what I have? Yes, is the answer. I both like what I have now and I would like you to be here. I was walking through the new passageway at King's Cross station and I suddenly thought of you together with the phrase 'perfect partner' and my eyes pricked with easy tears, the chin wobbling. Such a public place yet also a place where no one notices.

I came to see you the day after I got back and you were much better than when I left. You were up and dressed and sitting in the lounge, in the wing for the less well residents. I gave you your lunch but I'm not sure there was any spark of recognition from you to me. But you were laughing a bit and sort of chatty. I didn't stay that long. I wasn't ready for those emotions to be pulled just yet.

Getting up for my first day back at work I thought I no longer want to wear the blacks and greys that seem to make up my entire wardrobe. I spent a fortune on-line buying clothes in colours I normally ignore.

And I am still having dreams – I dreamed so much in Deia, usually about you being out of your care home and nowhere near as ill as you are now, but in those earlier stages and I'm confused about where you need to be. This dream on my return home was first in the care home, and there was a belligerent social worker berating me for not thinking enough about Irene's needs, why wasn't she being kept more active, and so on. I was stunned. Pam, the lovely qualified nurse was siding with me, saying, once the social worker had moved on, well we are doing the right things, what else can anyone expect? Then Irene was out of the home and we were somewhere or other, lots of people milling around. There was a dance floor and I said, 'Let's dance.' And of course I have new confidence now, as since you left in 2007 I have learnt to dance, can do a passable waltz, foxtrot or quickstep. You always despaired when you tried to teach me. I think I could never get it as you took the lead but didn't explain what I was meant to be doing. We never managed to dance together. Anyway, in my dream we took to the floor and, although initially you weren't sure what we were doing, I just took off, surprising even myself, and you followed. We swept round that floor doing a proper waltz, such that my legs were flowing, doing big long strides, and people were making way for us, two people dancing properly whereas they were just shuffling about. We glided round that floor as if we were one. Then I woke up. But I remember what it feels like to be dancing with you.

I saw the film *The Life of Pi* and it's a novel you taught once, long ago. What stays with this man called Pi, who endured over 200 days at sea in a small boat with a full-grown Bengal tiger, is that at the end of their journey, after bearing so much together, the tiger simply lopes into the forest and does not look back. He does not say goodbye. Pi thought they had a bond but the tiger was not aware of any such thing. It stung me. It hit me how cruel it is when something is left undone, unsaid.

It makes no difference to the love Irene and I had, which will endure anything, but it would have been complete if we could have done or said something before that forest enclosed you for good.

Things I'd Like to Tell You

I've read my first Mickey Spillane book. (I know! But I was in a hotel and there was nothing else to read.) Then, men were men, babes were babes, fairies were fairies, black folks were bartenders and maids, and corpses didn't talk.

Times have changed. There's so much you don't know.

You would be amazed now at the discussions about same sex marriage, not just civil partnerships; you don't know that there's a black man in the White House but you'd be delighted and you'd know that when he was born, black people did not have the vote. It's been as revolutionary for us. When you and I first met I'd just moved into the area as I'd got a job, and there was meant to be another person appointed to a parallel post. The woman who was favourite was turned down as the chair of the appointing panel thought she was too masculine. The job also provided free housing, as the warden of a student hostel, and the young women there might be in danger… I said nothing at the time – I needed the job. It wouldn't happen now – would it? And now there's a furious debate about same sex marriage – straight people falling out over it! Amazing. Straight people fighting for our rights. You were so happy that we were getting married, as you called it at our civil partnership, and then that we were married.

I finished our walk, all the way. Land's End to John o'Groats. I found out that I loved Cornwall and I've been back several times. You and I never explored it. I still cannot face the Lake District but I miss it and I will go – soon.

My lovely, big sister Penny has moved to Australia with her family, including her little grandkids who meant so much to me. It means I have no close family nearby. ('Oh no!' you'd say.) Three years now and yes, I do miss her like hell. But hey, I'm being a grown-up about it and there's always Skype. ('Not the same though, Rach,' you'd say.

'Oh come here. Let me give you a hug.')

I made that trip I always said I would when I was looking after you at home, that kept me going. I have been to the Arctic. I have seen polar bears.

I spent thousands of pounds on the ground floor of our house. I have knocked walls down. I have marked out on the ground the fact that it's just me there. I chose stuff I like. But you would love the wood burning stove. You always wanted one.

You have another generation added to your family in the shape of Eva, your nearly four-year-old great niece, and Edward, your nearly two-year-old great nephew. I'm sorry they will never get the benefit of your sense of fun or that you will never read them their bedtime stories. Everyone else is fine, just fine.

My work is stressful but it's OK. I don't have any plans to retire.

You would laugh, my love, but I've joined an evening class and I'm learning Japanese.

Love you baby. But then you know that.

The Year of 2013

In January I met with Meg, Brian's agent in London, in the new part of King's Cross station in one of those coffee places that is sort of open to the elements, or at least to the mass of commuters, but also sort of inside. We sat among others having a quick coffee and I felt relieved that we could not be emotional or even that personal in such an exposed place, not that I wanted to be with a stranger. She was very moved by the book draft. I was expecting her to say that my opus was really for private consumption and even if there was anything publishable it needed to be pared down from its 64,000 words. Not only was it publishable – it needed to be longer, for no books sell unless it is 100,000 words. I wanted to pick up her point, wondering about Joan Didion, C S Lewis and Julian Barnes who all have beautiful (and best-selling) slim volumes of their own griefly outpourings. But she knows the market. I saw a gap in the market for a book like the one I proposed, but she saw that as a sign that no one could get such books published. So I am two steps forward and one back in this marathon of writing, my confidence jilted and then boosted.

16 February 2013   Irene was so ill on Tuesday after a fit the day before. I had got annoyed for once, trying to feed her. I had to turn away as I wanted to force her mouth open, say Dammit, can't you? Open your mouth! Eat!

Today she was far better and I was surprised, as she was up and seated in the sunny, side lounge. Beautiful day, the sort on which we would by now be out on the hills.

I asked the name of the new resident, a little old lady sitting in the corner. Both staff looked at me a little alarmed. 'Why? Is she all right?' one asked. I said, 'Yes, fine.' She added, 'Oh, I ask because she throws things.' Her name is Mary. Little Mary, ulcerated legs, sitting quietly eating her porridge. I wanted her to throw something just so I could see what it was like.

Afterwards in the car park I bumped into a woman who visits Jack and, as I hadn't seen him, I asked if he was OK. 'Yes, just fast asleep.' We got into more than just an exchange of pleasantries. It turns out she is not his wife, as I thought, but his niece. Jack is 92. I thought him 10 years younger. I said I'd like to go to his funeral – she had brought it up, saying it was all paid for, it would be at St Mark's. It turns out his wife didn't want to know. Years before, she had left him at a hospital without telling the staff anything, so they were relieved to be in contact with this niece. The wife, according to the niece, had tried to keep all his money but they had managed to get some to pay for the funeral. He had been a teacher. She asked about Irene, asking who I was, a sister? I said no, partner, and she didn't flinch or show surprise. She was nice. Her sister who shared the visiting had just got oesophageal cancer. I got the impression she, the sister, would not be visiting from now on. She was pleased I wanted to go to the funeral whenever it happened, as there would be few others there. Jack had no children and they had lived down south. He had moved here to the home to be near the nieces, once his wife had disowned him. Jack had known the score when he was well enough, in the early days after his arrival, which I remember, about four years ago. Jack knew me, and always shakes my hand. When he first arrived I had conversations which sort of made sense. Now he looks at me quizzically and sometimes says a few words, but he always has a smile and looks at me with astonishingly piercing blue eyes.

The last week has been hard. I have missed Irene with an intensity that I thought had diminished. It has been her birthday and Valentine's Day and I have succumbed to that self-pity that says I will never meet her like, I will spend my days alone and that the best days are gone. I even descended into tears in front of my new manager, when at the end of a meeting I asked what the date was and she said, 'Why, it's Valentine's Day, how could you forget that?' I thought: I have not forgotten, I have bled all day, and then the easy tears came, my face crumbling into a redness and sorrow that I know I would hate if I saw myself in the mirror.

It seems that one drawback of the World Wide Web that is only just being recognised is that it's impossible to erase anything. It would be lovely to have recall of all the times we had. Or would it? There is so much I cannot remember. I know that forgetting is part of the human psyche – otherwise we might go mad. Those with hyperthymesia

– when they can recall what they were wearing on such and such a day in 1973 and what they said to whom – must be living a nightmare. They must have no space in their head for anything else but an overwhelming battery of memories. But it's also frightening when you have no recall whatsoever of having been somewhere, yet the objective facts say you were there. You have a photograph, or someone else swears they have a memory of it all.

But now I have my imagination, and they (who? neurologists, I suppose) reckon that imagination and memory share the same neural pathways, originate from the same parts of the brain. My brain's ability to forget is surely also connected to its ability to reconstruct, and also, to construct as if for the first time. So what's a memory and what's imagination? I know that I can remember how you looked and how you smiled but I also know that my imagination constructs these because often I can see you, aged 66, well and whole and laughing. That didn't happen but it's in my memory bank. Weird. It's another jump to thinking that it's real, and that way madness lies. But how or why do we remember certain things and not others? Some things stick in my mind and lots have been erased. Are they erased, or are they still there but I cannot recall them?

2 May 2013   1.15 in the morning. That was when you died. I knew you would die that night.

I knew you were not going to die the night before, though you fooled us into thinking you might. The staff thought so, and earlier I had dragged Gordon and Pauline in, apologizing, saying I don't know but I think we should go in, not being able to get in as the security code had come on the door. Gordon was perplexed, he hadn't yet cottoned on that 'making her comfortable' meant she was dying, that we were not even going to try to give you drinks or food. The GP was called out after dark and he said it could be a day or so or it could be a week. Leaving, I felt you would survive the night, and you did. You rallied in fact, though Pam the lovely in-charge said that people often rally before they die.

Earlier on the Tuesday I had watched you have a fit, the first I'd seen, even though you've had so many. You cannot keep the medication down. It was awful, ferocious, sudden, violent. Horrible to watch. You went a peculiar deep purple colour.

Then on Wednesday night I had to get to you, so I arrived at 8 in the evening. We had a few nice hours, didn't we? I didn't know what to expect, so I just sat and stroked your head, your arm, your hands. It was peaceful. You were moving your arms aimlessly, moving them slowly, partly as you didn't seem to know where to put them. You seemed semi-conscious, eyes skew-whiff, not really focusing. You are so thin, like a concentration camp victim. I have never seen anyone so thin. Your hips jut out. Your cheeks are hollowed. There are no muscles left anywhere.

After several hours, you turned your head – you were lying on your side. You were looking for me in the room. I came over to you, bending over really close. You spoke to me. You were not just making random sounds but telling me something in sounds, as that is all you have. You made sounds into sentences. There were three or four sentences of soft sounds. Then a big tear slowly rolled out of one eye. I replied. I said it's OK, it's all OK. And you were telling me everything. You were telling me what you could.

And I was stunned. How can someone who is so far gone, so semi-conscious, so near death, suddenly do something that has all the meaning in the world? It was not imagined, it was not romanticized; it was uncanny and it was real.

After that I decide to leave. Should I have stayed? I am a pragmatist; we had said all there was to say. My recovering broken ankle was painful, I was too tired. I needed to go. I didn't know how long it would be but I did know I was leaving you for the last time. I did want to be there for the end. But I wasn't. I can live with that. Would you have let go if I had been there? I did not want to prolong your agony. And you were in agony. It was awful to watch. Everyone has asked me if she was peaceful. I'm not sure what that means or how to answer.

Phone call at 1.20 am telling me you had just died.

Arranging your funeral. We found ourselves in the front room of what had once been a normal semi-detached house. Clever, as it had the feel of someone's living room, with living room proportions. It had two sofas, a couple of armchairs. But there were glass cabinets showing funeral products – have you thought about a nice urn for the ashes, what about a memorial plate? On the low coffee tables there were brochures for flowers, long sprays to fit neatly on top of a coffin.

I had not expected to be arranging the funeral so soon, when you had only been dead for 15 hours. But we were there, so we might as well have arranged it. The funeral director was a youngish man, made older by an abundance of excess weight, the sort of shape where his middle carried on southwards, leaving you wondering where his balls were. There was no sign. He was far more perfunctory than I had expected of a funeral director – kindly but too neutral, asking questions as if we might have been reporting an insurance claim. Later, when I met two others, I saw more of the depth of concern that you see in those programmes that enquire into 'unusual occupations' and film these saintly ordinary people going about their jobs of cleaning up other people's crap, or tenderly washing bodies, dead or alive. But our man for the time being was adequate. Gordon, Pauline and I had by chance intended to visit the crematorium that day to be sure it was what we wanted. Instead we went to a hotel nearby for lunch. We were really casing it as a possible venue for a funeral tea and indeed it turned out to be perfect, that side of the business run by a couple of twentysomethings and I thought that meant we'd get sandwiches with wholemeal instead of cotton-wool white. I decided the crematorium was OK – located in the dip of a valley, lots of trees, modern and bright, unlike the one nearer to us that was heavily embossed with religion. I had been there the week before for George's funeral and was reminded again of what a gloomy place it is, and set in a windy spot that caught all sorts of northern gusts that chilled. So before the end of the afternoon, when you had been dead for part of a night, a morning and an afternoon, we had decided where you would be cremated, and to where we retire to afterwards to meet and greet, and to talk about you, how we all knew you and what our connections were. Or are.

We had also decided what flowers, no car, except yours taking you to the crematorium, what coffin – plain ash, £385, the cheapest. You would have approved. Well, it's only going to get burnt, you'd say. I was surprised to find that wicker and cardboard were more expensive. No financial incentive to go green. I chose a lovely spray of flowers in yellow and blue; blue your favourite colour, irises as a reprise for my mother, Iris May. I made decisions as I often do about consumer choices – quickly. I realised I had never really thought about it all before, except that you and I would agree on the general principles – skimp on the things that don't matter so much (to us), like the coffin, but make sure there's lots of food.

5 May 2013   Miss you babe. I wish all this malarkey wasn't happening. Now I've got your funeral to organize. Yes, your funeral. Why did you leave this for me to do?

I almost wish there was something inside you that would cause an explosion. The undertakers ask all sorts of questions about implants. I mentioned your stapedectomy, the bit of Teflon in your ear. He looked at me as if I was deranged.

It didn't go down too well later either, when I took some clothes in. It had never occurred to me that you would need clothes. I had brought that top and trousers you bought once at the Great Yorkshire show, a cotton blue-checked shirt and matching blue trousers, cornflower blue. The funeral directors said any clothes had to be natural fibres and they carefully made out a receipt for them. You hardly fit those clothes any more. The undertaker said, 'Is that all?' the sub-text of which I took to mean, 'Don't you understand the meaning of dignity in death?' meaning, 'Where's the underwear?' So you are there with no underwear.

10 May 2013   Gordon and I came to visit you when you had been laid out in your coffin. The funeral director said in hushed tones that you were ready for us, as a butler might announce guests, as if you were sitting waiting. First we both came in to see you, and I was shocked. Then I left and Gordon spent some time with you. I don't know what he did in there and I didn't ask him.

When he came out, I went back in. I remember that I swore quite a lot and I spoke to you in a mutter of expletives, like bloody hell, bloody hell what have they done to you, Jesus Irene, what's happened, where have you gone. Then I calmed down a bit and looked at the coffin lid, studied the brass plate (is it brass?) with your name on it. And all the time expecting you to shift slightly, to shuffle, to move, any small movement. I took a photo of you, dead. I don't know if it's the done thing. It fits with the photos I took of you in the last days just before you died, a last one of me and you. You do look different dead, even though I thought you looked nearly dead in that last day or so. Really dead is different from being almost dead, the unimaginable pallor when the blood has finally stopped pumping.

You were the first corpse I'd seen. I kept waiting for you to breathe or to move slightly. I could hardly believe that you wouldn't. You were cold as a marble slab on a winter's day. I was shocked. I kissed your forehead and it was like kissing – well, cold marble. I had no idea it was our blood that keeps us so warm.

You looked – dead. I cannot believe I've got to my sixtieth year and have never seen a body before. You only just fit in the coffin. They have cocked one leg slightly and there were your bare feet. I didn't think about socks for you.

You don't make a pretty corpse my love. And I had to smile, among all the shock and expletives, at how I have survived you. You'd be mad; the rivalry of an old couple, one outliving the other. Ha! I won. If you were here, you would hit me. And we would laugh together.

It has helped to see you, really dead. I know it for a fact. There really is something complete about having the body there in front of you, knowing where your loved one's remains are. Completion.

You'd have loved the funeral. It was sort of understated but very affectionate and very emotional. I knew I didn't want a vicar. We had to have Bob Dylan, so they brought you in to the song 'Don't Think Twice It's Alright' and you went out to the final goodbye, into the flames, to Gracie Fields singing 'Wish Me Luck As You Wave Me Goodbye'. It brought a ripple of laughter as that song started up and it was just you; I could imagine you singing along to the chorus when she goes, 'Whoo hoo hoo, whoo hoo hoo, whoo hoo hoo', in place of a chorus.

It all went beautifully and I was pleased. I had ordered 60 orders of service and we were woefully short. If the place was full, and people said it was, it seats 120 people. It seems that everyone came.

We were lucky as the funeral before yours was short, the few attendees scuttling back to their cars as we arrived, half an hour early. Maybe it was an old person with no relatives and, I imagined, a sad end to a lonely life. There were certainly no emotions that I could see amongst the fleeing few. So we had time to gather and time to be ushered in before our allotted time. Everyone arriving, hushed, everyone knowing the code of behaviour at a funeral. Your name was lit up on the board proclaiming the order of funerals. In neon. Startling.

I took my place on the front row and after a look around for nieces and nephews who had hidden at the back instead of being near us, not knowing the form at funerals and where the proper place for family is, I turned to face the front, knowing that I could not afford to meet anyone's eye or, really, to save them the fearful look in mine. So you arrived without me really seeing you, to Bob Dylan, in the coffin I had chosen. I had wanted you to come in to the strains of the *Arrival of the Queen of Sheba* and for the first words of the celebrant to be, 'Irene always did think she was a queen' but I knew it wouldn't come off, that it was a private joke. So instead there you were: don't think twice it's alright.

And your friends did you proud; first your brother giving a tribute to his little sis, a loving older brother who cracked up as he neared the end, and being a man, berated himself for that for the rest of the day. And Jean, telling stories of you in your twenties, of how much fun and laughter there was. Then Barbara read a poem that is loved in the family, and was read at Daniels' funeral:

Say not the struggle nought availeth,
The labour and the wounds are vain,
The enemy faints not, nor faileth,
And as things have been, things remain.

If hopes were dupes, fears may be liars;
It may be, in yon smoke concealed,
Your comrades chase e'en now the fliers,
And, but for you possess the field.
For while the tired waves, vainly breaking,
Seem here no painful inch to gain
Far back through creeks and inlets making
Came, silent, flooding in, the main,

And not by eastern windows only,
When daylight comes, comes in the light,
In front the sun climbs slow, how slowly,
But westward, look, the land is bright.

Nice touch, eh? But westward, look, the land is bright. You'd have loved that and I can imagine your dad reading it out, with his slight lisp because of his funny teeth that would have been fixed by a free NHS if he'd been born 60 years later. Then Pauline reading her bit, also saying what a privilege it was to have you as her funny, gangly, sister-in-law, as a prelude to her reading my letter to you. She read it beautifully of course, possibly the only tough cookie who could get through it without cracking up. I had written it about a year ago and didn't change a thing when it came to it. It said all I wanted and needed to say and I said it in public. I did worry for a day or so if it was too emotional but where else was I going to say it? So I did. Or at least, Pauline did. Then a song I wanted, which was Eva Cassidy singing 'I Know You By Heart' because it summed us up and told a story. I did know you by heart, a double entendre, knowing you by heart and our hearts leading the way. And you are still here beside me every day.

Midnights in Winter
The glowing fire
Lights up your face in orange and gold.
I see your sweet smile
Shine through the darkness
Its line is etched in my memory.

So I'd know you by heart.

Mornings in April Sharing our secrets
We'd walk until the morning was gone.
We were like children
Laughing for hours
The joy you gave me lives on and on.

'Cause I know you by heart.
I still hear your voice
On warm Summer nights
Whispering like the wind.

You left in Autumn
The leaves were turning
I walked down roads of orange and gold.
I saw your sweet smile
I heard your laughter
You're still here beside me every day.

'Cause I know you by heart,
'Cause I know you by heart.
Then there was not much more to be said, so the celebrant announced

that Irene was now off on her final journey and that's when Gracie Fields joined us and it was a lovely break in the sadness and tension. And then I had to turn to face all those people, as the crematorium has the exit at the back. I could look at no one but I stood outside at the bottom of the steps and greeted everyone, thanked them all for coming. Everyone said what a wonderful service it was and I think they all meant it. It was rather beautiful and people seemed surprised, but for me it was the obvious thing to do – just get people to talk about Irene and make it all fit in the time. The time management was everything and I had lain awake at night thinking about it. How odd that we conduct funerals in this way. I thought of all the funerals I'd been at in Africa where the whole thing takes the time it takes – there, no one would dream of putting time constraints around it, cramming it into a predetermined 'slot'. Here it's choreographed down to parts of minutes, timed to perfection, bits cut out as they cannot be fitted in. I had wanted some Wordsworth, perhaps even some Joyce Grenfell, more poetry. But in a way, a 40-minute slot, as our abrupt funeral director had pointed out, was enough. And so to the hotel for the bun fight.

All those people in one place, your life measured out, not in coffee spoons but in a procession of faces from each part of your life and each era.

It only just occurred to me last night, in bed, nursing an increasingly sore throat, that I could be resentful of all the tragedy that has occurred over the last ten years and that I might have a grievance for having to put up with so much for a decade. It hasn't really occurred to me to be resentful.

7 August 2013 People ask me what I'm going to do with your ashes. I say that I will keep them so that we can be scattered somewhere together one day. I don't go so far as to say that for now they are next to my bed, our bed, in the wooden box that was one of the few things you took from your parents' house after they had died. It's a solid box, not valuable but of some meaning to you. It fits your ashes well.

I miss you.

I have to repeat it: You died on 2 May. Not so long ago really. Three months and five days actually. You don't know that you've died so

I need to tell you these things. But you seemed to know you were dying. I wrote to the lovely woman who I had hoped would do your funeral. (She couldn't do the service in the end as she'd moved to Brighton – 'it was very special and privileged work, but I am happy not to have death in my life every day' she replied.) Anyway this is what I told her. I haven't told many people because, well, the telling somehow diminishes it. I couldn't say it without cracking up and also I don't want to see people's expressions of disbelief. I wrote this earlier, but this is what I told her:

I was with Irene until a couple of hours before she died. I knew she would die that night. I was with her, just the two of us. And at one point, even though she'd been semi-conscious and seemingly unaware, she looked around – she was so weak she could hardly lift her head, but she definitely looked for me in the room and then said something, not just sounds but as if she was speaking words and then one tear came out of her eye. She was trying to tell me something even at such a late stage. Then I left shortly after as that seemed all there was to say. It seems now like something I might have made up or imagined.

She believed me. 'Thanks for sharing that with me Rach – I am so glad you were with her. I am sure you didn't imagine it. All kinds of things happen when someone rallies their last strength, and it was obviously you she would turn to and communicate with. The phrase that came to my mind when I met with you both was that she turned to you like a flower to the sun. It doesn't have to be verbal. Such experiences are to be treasured.'

She apologized for not being able to conduct the service. 'I am truly sorry for that – I would have really liked to have helped you in this small way. I was very much moved by meeting you and Irene and I will never forget it. Particularly the way she smiled when she first saw you – it seemed to me there was still so much love there between you, in spite of all.'

I am always taken aback at how other people can see what I know.

I miss you more now than I ever thought, as if the dementia years have fallen away and I am left with the old you and my imagined you, as you would have been without Alzheimer's.

I have no wish to return to any world of Alzheimer's. I do not miss the care home or any of the people there. It was a demented decade, enough for anybody. Our Dementia Decade. My only regret is that I wasn't there when you died. I'd heard from someone that often people choose to die when they're alone, hanging on when there's someone there. Maybe that's why I left. I will have to live with this now.

I thought missing you would diminish but that doesn't appear to be the deal.

I've just had a letter from the Department of Work and Pensions. I perked up to see that they had followed up your opted out contributions and that I was owed something. I then read that the amount would be £2.19 a week.

£8.76 a month sounds more and it's a whole £113.88 a year. And in a decade it's £1,138.80!

25 September 2013 I've been shredding old credit card statements. Sometimes they show the mundane purchases, petrol at our local garage, a supermarket shop, and other times they let me know when we did things – the Hotel Tudor in Tewkesbury, where we arrived so late that I bargained with the young man at the desk and told him what we'd pay; another in the Scottish borders. It told me when we had done that part of our Land's End to John o'Groats walk, which I was grateful for, as I had forgotten the year. I enjoy the act of shredding, a quick burr of electric blades and a copious pile of white paper worms. I put them in one of the black compost bins, where they will be chomped by real worms, and where they will bed down and disappear within a surprisingly short space of time. I won't think of a shredded life; they are just documents.

I've started to worry slightly about how people will find my important documents. I mean, when I die. I've put my new will on the noticeboard in my study, pinned in its old fashioned-looking envelope.

Brian is producing his play. He has a group of professional actors, five of them, two playing you and me. It's weird, of course, and I cried when my character started to read out the lines that I had written. It's like watching animated facsimiles but there are times when it doesn't seem like me and you at all. I showed them the DVD of you in 2007 when you so poignantly talked about how you used to act. I nearly lost it when we started it up, a great well of a sob that could have gone one way or another – subside or sweep me away. It did the former, and I relaxed, stood at the back, relieved that I didn't need hugs and sympathy; that I could keep it together. I don't want the attention. And there you were, in our garden only a couple of months before the crash through the ice. You did that little shimmy, the little wave to the camera. And of course the actors laughed ruefully when you said 'I couldn't do it now, you have to keep it all up here', tapping on your head. You'd have loved to have played the role yourself – but if you could have done there'd have been no need for a play about Irene and Rach's story of early onset dementia.

I felt a certain thrill going behind the scenes at the West Yorkshire Playhouse, needing a security swipe card to access those areas normally closed to me. I felt I had to wear a black T-shirt and try to look a little arty. I don't think I need have worried as all the actors seem perfectly normal and if you had seen us all at the table over lunch you never would have suspected that the gaggle of middle aged men and women were, in fact, actors. About half have personal experience of dementia – fathers, a mother – of an experience with a loss, like the one who will play Cindy, who looked after her husband for six years after he had cancer, a stroke, two heart attacks.

And now you really are gone. You don't know that you died in the middle of the night, 2 May 2013, aged 66. You would have had no idea how old you were.

I'd have loved to be able to tell you about the funeral, how special it was.

My heart sank knowing I had to get out of bed and go into Leeds, meet the actors. It was that same sense of depression, a low, that has hung over me for months. Can't I just stay in bed a bit longer, not have to face it all just yet? That feeling has left me recently and I've been more enthusiastic, prising myself from my warm duvet. Facing it all again, the past, when all I want to do is embrace the future. Dealing with all the emotion, the loss, the regrets; the memory of your smile, your laugh, your eyes loving me. Too much. And I have a life I'm enjoying – this month.

August was awful – have gone from famine to feast in terms of happiness and hope. August was dark, too much on my own resources, feeling sorry for myself, and missing you with a keening emptiness. Going back to work properly has helped so much, far more than I ever thought it would – doing something productive, being with people, having something outside of myself. Suddenly the loss doesn't seem to be foregrounded but has slipped into a shadowy background which doesn't intrude.

September, that time of a new term, of a not-so-subtle change in the feel of the air, of striking out again.

26 September 2013   You speak to me from beyond.

Seamus Heaney died a few weeks ago so I found a copy of his poems on your/our shelves. It's old – his *Collected Poems 1965-1975*. There's one called 'Poem for Marie'. At the end you have written, in your idiosyncratic, unmistakable handwriting, in pencil: 'Leaving the imperfect child behind: washing away sense of incompleteness in the past'.

You always did have to explain poems to me.

6 October 2013   My life is pretty good right now. It's October, the season of mists and mellow fruitfulness. It was always our month and I drift back to when I was 26 years old, falling in love with you under autumn skies, hearing the sound that only kicking through piles of golden leaves can make. It's the first of our anniversaries – 22 October – that you won't actually be here. I had never seen a dead body before yours, let alone touched one. How privileged I have been, not to have been in a situation where dead bodies were likely to be seen – never been in a war zone, unlike you, in Addis Ababa, stepping over dead bodies in the street on your way to work.

There's an abundance of fruit in this year of abundant sunshine and our freezer is full of plums and apples, plus more to pick on the trees. And our middle-class circle has embarked on its autumnal round of gift relationships, taking bags of pears, apples, courgettes, a few remaining beans, to neighbours, colleagues and friends. And in this new term there's an abundance of culture, literature festivals, concerts, as all the (again, predominantly middle class) reconnect after their summers. So this weekend alone I have met Erwin James, seen William Dalrymple and Germaine Greer and been to hear the Tchaikovsky Symphony Orchestra of Radio Moscow.

As usual, I pick and sift through what I'm taking in, distilling bits that relate to you, us, to my experience, memory and loss. I wonder when I'll stop doing that, but all around there seem to be things said, overheard, read, that are relevant. Maybe that's because really all life is about memory, love and loss. So, reading the concert notes, I read that Tchaikovsky's pizzicato in his Fourth Symphony is meant to represent melancholia, and he himself wrote: 'The melancholy of a long procession of old memories gone by. The recollection of the past is sad because it has gone, but sweet because it was pleasurable.' And he describes Fate as an 'Inevitable force which checks our aspirations towards happiness before they reach their goal…This force is inescapable and invincible. There is no other course but to submit and inwardly lament'. I remember you explaining once the pure meaning of tragedy – that it's overused and should really only mean those occasions when something really was inevitable, inescapable. Poor Tchaikovsky, getting married to please his father and then botching his own suicide. I wonder how much more he went on to write after that, how much would have been lost had he been successful. And of course I am also bowled over by the music, that rolling refrain of the first movement of Rachmaninov's Third Piano Concerto and the turmoil of the rest. The strings of the Russian orchestra are immense – I count over 60 musicians in the string section alone, and it makes me realise that my life is suffused with shards of happiness, like sitting in dappled sunlight – or is it dappled shade? The dapples of sunlight have got bigger.

And we have been creating our own bit of theatre, you and I. The play has had its first public airing. Everyone asks if it's weird listening to my own words read out, or seeing myself portrayed on stage. It kind of is and it kind of isn't. There will always be a lot of it that is purely private, that no one except you and I will ever know. I do not need to explain us to anyone; I do not need to impress or try to give the truth of it all. So really anything else is a facsimile and the intention is not to be faithful to our story – it's not a re-enactment. Rather, it's about airing a story of dementia, what it's like, how it feels. And the script certainly does that. The story intertwines me and Irene, and another couple where the husband has Alzheimer's. He, his wife and daughter make up the five characters.

One of my contacts in the Alzheimer's world said at the end that she had sat through lots of plays about dementia, but that this one captured it the best. She and another colleague sat in floods of tears at the end. So did lots of others. I felt responsible for all the weeping. The woman next to me often had her face in her hands and at one point was trying to breathe calmly and slowly. I was worried she might be having a cardiac incident. And Jean cried and cried; later she said she'd not cried that much while Irene was ill and then had had to keep herself together to read at the funeral. And me? Well, by the Friday read-through I was interested in how the script had progressed and could put emotions on hold while my brain took over. There was only one point that caught me enough to bring tears – when the father, who has not known his daughter, suddenly says to her: 'You are a beautiful girl,' after she has just lamented how much she would love his advice about her future partner.

So, the play is done. Now the aim is to get it to a proper audience, not just a few invited people, and to get it to the stage, not just a read-through. In response to the question 'Is there anything else that you would like to see incorporated into the play?', our lovely friend Jim wrote on the feedback form: 'The saddest facet for me is the growing separation, the violence (apparent) of the anger and aggression, the sense that your loved friend is an "emptying vessel" and will eventually vanish without goodbye on either side. I feel this was not fully expressed'. And Jean wrote that she'd like to see 'More about the drama and poetry in Irene's life'.

10 October 2013   An item came on the radio news as I was waking up – scientists have announced that they have taken a major step forward in treating Alzheimer's. I burst into tears. Too late for you.

Later they had a scientist on and she was tentative, nowhere near the excitement generated by the press. It seems they have turned a scientific corner and have identified the process which can be targeted by a compound which will halt the brain damage caused by whatever agent is responsible. And of course it's poor hapless mice that have been worked on so far. But I do have to be glad – if in the future it will help even a few, it will be worth it.

I thought about Jim's comment about a growing separation, of the vessel becoming empty. I thought about the terror of forgetting your background, all the 'known' falling away; daily life suddenly full of the most horrible pitfalls into which you regularly fall. All tacit understanding of what is usual or right disappears, the everyday is suddenly – or slowly – treacherous. In the place of the ongoing flow of daily routine comes uncertainty, flashes of the known but mostly disorientation. And of course daily life changes for we carers too and those incidents of violence, anger and aggression become the new normal, aspects of life to be managed.

Married life for those who have been together so long falls into an easy familiarity, a shared narrative that makes sense of it all. But that shared narrative of daily life disappears: I had no idea really what you were going through and I could no longer share my day. Your days were full of things like failing to understand the story line of a TV drama and so stomping off to bed, blaming the post-modern playwright. Later on, I had no idea that at times you did not know who I was. It's only later that that makes sense of your fear of being in a strange car with a stranger. So – if this scientific breakthrough is what it is, I will also shed tears of joy, not just of disappointment.

19 October 2013   Of course I'm not always unhappy. When I start to write this journal, this book, whatever it is, I'm drawn back and then I get upset, have a good weep. Life isn't like that all the time. I guess I can appear to my friends as if it's life as normal – almost – and I too get on with stuff, go to a film, go to hear interesting people speak, have dinner with friends. A few weekends ago someone I'd met on PinkSofa came to stay. There was no chemistry – I knew at first sight, but hey, I'm trying.

It was with huge relief that I put her on the train, waved cheerily as she looked for me through the window, smiles all round. And back to our house, back to normality, somehow, you and me again, or at least me and the absence of you. I think I've decided to give this internet dating lark a miss, not to renew my membership, as it's so odd a process – the expectation building up after you seem able to chat so well on the phone, and then the heart-sinking moment (and it is a moment) that you actually meet and realise that not only is there no chemistry, but that there never will be any chemistry. We got along well enough, managed to find conversation, things to do together. But it was all bittersweet too: if you were here I wouldn't be doing this, so it's the biggest reminder that, indeed, you are not here.

It would of course have been different had we clicked; then, the two nights and a long day would have flown by instead of presenting an hour-by-hour set of problems as to how to get through them. There's no way of knowing whether there will be any chemistry before you meet. And what is that indefinable chemistry anyway?

So I am back in my village routine, calling in to my chum in the village whose husband has Alzheimer's. Three days ago, his son from his first marriage died suddenly at the age of 50; Carrie and their daughter are in a quandary whether to tell him or not. My advice is not to, and they are both gravitating to that. There's nothing to help you through these practical and ethical dilemmas except gut feeling and accumulated wisdom. If they told him, he would forget, and go through the agony of being told the news as if for the first time again and again. I felt for them. Then, as is often the way, a number of helpers turned up – their cleaner and then the physio's assistant, to check on Noel's state of mobility, and I left. A rainy walk home, and fleeting memories of when we too were in that phase, strangers turning up to assess, to help, and all your real feelings get put on hold for the duration of their stay.

9 November 2013   I so often have the feeling that I am merely passing time; it's not unpleasant but I am merely passing the time.

I wouldn't mind so much now if I were to shuffle off this mortal coil. I no longer have the horror of an early death, and anyway you might not know about it. I would offer myself in place of the young mother with two kids if we were captured by kidnappers. I would do the *Tale of Two Cities* swap – 'tis a far, far better thing and all that. I am too squeamishly cowardly ever to take my own life and anyway life's not that dire, although I have sometimes stepped into the shoes of those who do commit that act and I've thought it quite rational. But it is also, in my book, an immoral act. I could not do that to my remaining parent, siblings, friends. It seems an overly dramatic response and anyway I am nothing if not eternally optimistic. I find it hard to think that my best times are over. And sometimes I feel scared of how few spring seasons there might be to see in, all that wonderful new growth of an English May.

I knew 2013 was going to be a year. I knew in February that I could not carry on without a break. I was sent one. You know that the earth of Africa is red but it seems all the more red when you are sitting on it, all focus gone except for that trained on your ankle, which is bulging oddly and you know that you cannot stand. You wave to some workmen and they wave back but carry on with their work. Eventually a man appears from the bush. It's 7.15 in the morning, people are starting to go to work. You think it's a good idea to try to stand, God knows why, so you place your dangling foot squarely on the earth with your hands, grab this man's skinny waist. Not a good idea and you collapse again on the road in pain, crying out. And a long story cut short means a dislocated ankle that is broken in three places. Ghana's Day of Independence, 6 March, so staff have to be called away from the morning's parade and celebrations to tend to a European who slipped on a road while walking before work. The man, I'm not sure of his actual job title, pulls my foot back into place and with his wonderful use of words, says, beaming broadly, 'I'm caressing your foot,' as I lay flat out on a gurney. I've only had two paracetamol but I can't say it's too excruciating. I am now undislocated, but I have my break.

Then I am back in England, my West African work cut short, eight days in hospital whilst they insert a plate and pins and then another six weeks of non-weight bearing. They note that I live alone; the OT talks me through it all as if I've never considered how I might manage. It is hard but I become a dab hand at hoisting myself around, on my bum, using my arms, setting it all up so I can eat, wash, sleep. Friends rally round of course and I have the most sociable time in years, new faces every night coming armed with recipes and ingredients.

Seven months on, I am back in Ghana, I have visited the spot where I fell so swiftly and with such dramatic effect. It's six months, two large scars, one death away. The kind hotel owner suggested he take me there in a golf cart. He took me to the hospital when it happened. He's delighted to see me again. We drive up to the spot, my colleagues in tow, all merry at being driven around in an electric golf cart. The road has now been tarred and looks and feels different. Now there are no small pebbles like glass marbles to slip on, only a spanking new driveway that leads up to houses being built. The road gives out at the tree line and the land starts to rise even more steeply. It was a bit of a slope where I fell, but nothing more than that of my daily commute, the hill in my village to catch the train every morning. Freak accident.

I am incredibly nervous and decline to get out of the golf cart, seeing the view from under the frill of the cart's canopy. The shock of the fall somehow still seems to be in my body, as well as in my head. I have to explain the English saying of 'laying a ghost' to my Ghanaian colleagues.

The novelist Julian Barnes was married for the same time as Irene and me. Then his wife died. He writes,

Early in life, the world divides crudely into those who have had sex and those who haven't. Later, into those who have known love, and those who haven't. Later still – at least, if we are lucky (or, on the other hand, unlucky) – it divides into those who have endured grief, and those who haven't. The divisions are absolute; they are tropics we cross.

My break slowed me down enough that your death didn't hit me in full gallop, just at more of a canter. It meant I could give you my full attention, not also juggling work. That had already been taken care of. I was out of it. Julian Barnes makes the observation that 'We grieve in character'. Obvious but worth stating. Like him, I too suddenly became acutely aware of what it's like to lose your life's companion, in his words again, 'The heart of my life; the life of my heart'. I knew of it, of course, of what it might mean to lose your life's mate, but now I knew it. And all I can say, pathetically, when someone asks how I'm doing, is, 'Well, it's very profound losing your life partner,' rubbing it in, maliciously, for those who have not yet crossed that tropic but are terrified of it, and likewise, maliciously for those who have not known true love and probably never will. My words shut them out, which is what I intend.

And I find comfort in his words as he echoes, and says so much more eloquently, what I would have liked to have said. Barnes writes:

I do not believe I shall ever see her again. Never, see, hear, touch, embrace, listen to, laugh with; never again wait for her footstep, smile at the sound of an opening door, fit her body into mine, mine into hers. Nor do I believe we ever will in some dematerialised form. I believe dead is dead. Some think grief a kind of violent if justifiable self-pity; some that it is merely one's own reflection in death's eye; others say it's the survivor they feel sorry for, because they're the one going through it, whereas the lost loved one can no longer suffer. Such approaches try to handle grief by minimising it – and doing the same with death. It's true that my grief is self-

directed – look what I have lost, look how my life has been diminished – but it is more, much more, and has been from the beginning, about her: look what she has lost, now that she has lost life. Her body, her spirit; her radiant curiosity about life. At times it feels as if life itself is the greatest loser, the true bereaved party, because it is no longer subjected to that radiant curiosity of hers.

He solved the issue of whether to carry on or not, not by backing away from the goriness of it but by realising that, if he died, she would die again too, as he now carried all the memories for both of them.

As I write this, there's a hornbill sitting a few yards away outside my balcony, so close that through the small binoculars that were yours (mine being the big ones) I can see every feather, the marks on its huge bill, its shaggy legs. If I wasn't here I wouldn't be seeing it. So yes there are good times but they are a bit like a consolation prize.

He (Julian) ponders the difference between grief and mourning. 'Grief makes your stomach turn, snatches the breath out of you, cuts off the blood supply to the brain; mourning blows you in a new direction.' Grief, he suggests, is a state whereas mourning is a process. Sometimes you come out of that state – maybe that's part of the mourning process. Then sometimes here it comes again, hitting you in the solar plexus, bowling you off your feet. Like when I was swimming the Salford Quays Big Swim mile, my strategy for getting fit again after The Break – suddenly at the half-way mark I heard my name being called by my friend Kate, cheering me on, and it hit me with the force of a small tsunami that it should have been you cheering me on, and that you never will, except in my head. And I cried tears into the water of the Manchester Ship Canal, had to pull myself together. I agree that dead is dead. Yet I talk to you all the time, tell you things, ask you what to do.

Julian Barnes only had 37 days (and so did his wife Pat Kavanagh) to get used to the knowledge that she was dying. At least I had more warning. I almost see 29 August, the day you left home for good, as more of a death. 2 May was a shadow death but also the real death. Six years, almost, between those dates. And you appear in dreams. The anti-malaria tablets always seem to make me dream more – not only me; colleagues recognise it too. You are there of course, and the recurring theme is that you are well enough to be out and about, seeming normal, and I have to puzzle out why you are with me, yet you needed, earlier, to be in a home. How has this happened? Do I need to break it to you that you have to go back? Yet you seem OK, a bit eccentric, true, but capable of living outside. So do we just carry on as normal? It is always unresolved when I wake up, but it's lovely having that feeling of your being near, even if it's a dream. You've been there, there's a trace of you.

I have literally crossed the tropic and there's a tropical thunderstorm going on outside. And you feel as distant as the thunder rolling around. I cannot catch up with you.

Another dream: I have to catch a plane, I'm going somewhere for a few days for an important meeting. I arrive in Manchester at the airport there but at the terminal it's all changed and not how I remember. There's no one to tell me where to go, just some vague sense that I have to be somewhere else. I ask someone and she is rude, telling me to look on the airline website. I start to say that I don't have a laptop handy, and then two other employees enter and apologise, saying that the unhelpful employee has learning difficulties. I am pushed along, as they don't know either where I have to report, so I wander into another building that used to be a separate check-in hall for a budget airline but it's been turned into a restaurant. The attendants there are helpful when I show them a map I've acquired with an asterisk next to a civic building where I think I'm meant to check in; then I realise that I didn't exactly see anyone tell me that and maybe the scrawled star on the map is for an entirely different purpose, made by someone else. So I wander back to my friends – there's Irene and three other friends. We have time to kill (we think) and we are exploring an historic building. I suddenly realise I barely have time to catch my flight and still don't know where to go. Instead of a pert suitcase with smart work clothes inside, I've packed a large rucksack with nothing of much of use inside. I think I can buy an outfit at the airport – if only I could find it in time. I need to rush, so I call Irene, who by now has gone on ahead and is happily waiting to explore the upper floors of something like a belfry. She is with our friends. I call a goodbye and she cheerily stoops down across the bannister to give me a kiss, me standing on the lower staircase. She is happy whereas I'm the one who is anxious, confused, frustrated. She seems unaware that I am actually disappearing for a while – she is keen to get on with the immediate task, seeing what's around the very next corner. I wake up still having not found where I'm heading…

I am back in Accra, staying just one night before I catch another plane, at the home of Ghanaian friends I have known literally for a lifetime. It's been a while since I was here and things have changed. Their once distinctively splendid home has been overtaken by those of the newer posh homes of other, wealthier, younger Ghanaians. It's now bounded by a dual carriageway where once there had merely been a main arterial. The airport has encroached and Burma Camp looks, on the outside at least, more corporate. Inside, their house seems gloomy, there are more smudge marks on the white walls, the huge sofas where you could comfortably seat 20 people, are more faded; the white plastic around the light switches now grimy with finger marks. But the saddest is to see the father, still majestic but now felled, like a mighty tree. He is in pain, a slipped disc; I get the impression he has hardly moved from his bedroom for the last two years. He receives me there, a man used to directing the conversation but glad of some stimulating discussion. We talk of Ghanaian politics and I can't help taking in the settled dust, the old telephone alongside his new mobile, the bottles men use to urinate in, the bolsters, the towels and other signs of an invalided soldier.

For indeed he was a soldier, a very eminent one, once leading the UN Peace Corps Forces in the Lebanon, and I remind him that one of the most exciting stories I ever heard as a child was from him. It was 1966 and he was telling us how he'd been woken up at gun point, given us a vivid picture of a young officer in a narrow bed, a revolver inches away, those plotting the coup wanting to make sure that there would be no counter-coup from those military supporting their President, Kwame Nkrumah. And we talk of how Ghana might have been different if Nkrumah had not been ousted but of how at least there is stable government, and from that all good things could, and were, flowing. I am suddenly choked with emotion, as we talk of my mum, dead nearly a decade, and of the sacrifices he and his wife made to give their children a good education, when it was regarded as the only thing to do to send children abroad. Now six of the eight are part of the diaspora, in good jobs as lawyers, dentists in the Caribbean, North America, but somehow unsettled, and I wish they were home – partly for the sake of their parents, who suddenly seem lonely, and partly for their own sakes, to be part of a motherland from which they have been away for most of their lives. I want to say come home, be a family. I hope to meet one of the eight home-based children, but hear that he and his wife have just left for the States.

And here is a man who seems to have given up on life, the party long past its best. The living room is full of pictures of him in full uniform, posing with those familiar key global political figures from the 1970s who also tried to bring about world peace: Henry Kissinger, Kurt Waldheim, the handsome King of Jordan. He has had an eminent career, his once glamorous wife, the beautiful companion and also a driving force not just on the domestic front. There are still all the citations, letters of thanks from bodies such as the UN, framed and filling the walls, some of them recent. Their accents could be mistaken as British; his delivery has gravitas. I had been afraid to ask of him when I arrived; people on the outside had enquired, saying it had all gone quiet. But then she had said we should go upstairs to see Big Daddy I was both relieved and apprehensive. The houseboy, a lithe young man of about 17 who pads around silently in bare feet and who brings us beer, calls him Daddy. I call him by what I have known him as since childhood, Big Alex. To the community he is Uncle Ato. He is also a Lieutenant General, all versions of the same man. He now has to ring a bell when he wants a glass of water. He could have an operation but he is afraid of it further damaging his back. On the wall of the corridor outside his room there is a framed shield with the words 'Yield to Nothing'.

Downstairs she fills me in on all the family news and I get lost in a welter of grandchildren; we talk all the time on the phone she says. But I feel sad for them all somehow, faded glory and loved ones far away. I tell her all my family news too, the happiness and the sorrows. The full weight of the past – of what had been and what might have been – make me want to weep. It's not just about Irene, but I know too that the moment is coming where I will be asked about her. She has been in this house and, given the Ghanaian skills of social memory and the custom of courtesy and hospitality, I know she will be enquired after. And I know too that given the deep religion, the homophobia and the African aversion to same sex relationships that I cannot say what Irene really meant to me or what her death signifies. So I know that I have to get through telling them without breaking down, without tears. And, practised as gay people usually are at hiding our most deeply felt sense of who we are, somehow I manage it. I say that she died, this year in fact; a terrible shame, early onset Alzheimer's, in a home for the last six years. Somehow I manage not only to blink away the forming tears, swallow the pain in my throat, but also to take control of the conversation, and we move to the now, the present. There is more than 50 years of history with us, and we pick up where we left off, as you do with people you have known a long time. It's very special to be here.

The next morning I am sweating, the house warm and the heat only dispersed by a ceiling fan. I have been used to the fierce blasted cold of air conditioned offices. When I return in the afternoon from my errands, Daddy's door remains resolutely shut. I don't feel I have any permission to go there without his wife opening the way. A closed room, a great man inside. Other people, too, end up in sad places; we can't know what those closing years hold for us.

As ever, books help, and I'm reading *The Music Room* by William Fiennes, the book named for the room where his mother went to practice, playing to get away from it all. He was brought up in a castle, and it's a memoir of his childhood. Are all people called Fiennes posh and are they all related? It's really about his brother, who, like him, would have developed into an interesting, educated, employable young man had he not had such terrible epileptic seizures as a small child that his brain was damaged. Instead, this brother, Richard, grew to be beyond the coping capabilities of the family so he lived part of the time in a home, but also spent time at the family home, where he alternated between being violent, or on the verge of rage such that the household was kept in a state of tension, or being calmly obsessive and occasionally outrageously happy, such as when his football team, Leeds United, did well.

It all makes me wonder if Irene's own mood swings, the sudden frenzies before she went into care, can be explained by actual brain damage, rather than something more psychological, like fear. When she was in the care home for those last five years, she had any number of seizures. The staff would ring me, or not, depending on who was on duty. She was on strong epilepsy drugs before she died. It's how she broke her ankle, twice, in the home, and she had some fits that lasted minutes, others parts of minutes. It probably led to more lasting damage, as it had with Richard. He became prone to sudden violence, was asked to leave his care home and ended up being back at the castle for a year. William once came across his father standing silently with his hand pressed on to the stone of the old fortress that was their home. He asked him what he was doing and his father replied, 'I'm asking the house to give me strength'.

I only saw Irene have a fit once, in the few days before she died. It was a short one, maybe seconds, but it was still harrowing and I realised I was holding my breath. It was over before I could call for help. Anyway, what help could she have needed? I always knew when she was building up to one though, and now I can't recall exactly why. Maybe she wouldn't want the chocolate that she usually devoured, maybe she just seemed different. So when I was told, maybe half a day later, I wasn't surprised. They – the staff – were clearly a bit perplexed by the fits. It seems not everyone has them but it makes sense to me that if your brain is being eaten away it will affect the electrical circuitry just as, if a seaside bungalow is crumbling over an eroding cliff, there will be bare wires hanging out amid the jagged bits of masonry. Fiennes' memoir is punctuated by terrifying accounts of experiments from past centuries where surgeons removed parts of a patient's skull to expose the brain and then applied electrical currents. Patients reported all sorts of effects, such as hearing music. Nothing is reported of what happened to the patients afterwards but I guess we are to be grateful to these butcher surgeons for giving us an understanding of the electrical currents that make us what we are.

There's a passage where William talks about how this is what his brother has always seemed like to him, unaware that there could have been a different course for his big brother. He writes:

I knew my brother wasn't like other people, and I was starting to understand that this was because there were scars in his brain, behind his forehead. But I couldn't think of Richard's personality as a set of symptoms; I couldn't think of his character as a manifestation of disease. That would have implied the existence of an ideal healthy Richard my brother was an imperfection of, a dream-Richard this actual person couldn't measure up against. But there wasn't any other Richard.

I realise that I do have an ideal Irene, growing old disgracefully, without Alzheimer's, the Irene in my head, the Irene who turns to me suddenly and says, 'Oh, I do love you! But it is just a dream-Irene. And also I realise that her life is indistinguishable from the diseased state she grew into, that that was her, it shaped her, became her – there was no other. There is no other Irene. She was the disease, and the disease was her. It was her life, the Alzheimer's was an integral part of her, she did not exist without it. It's a dead-end, there is no parallel universe where she exists, happy and content, exploring a belfry. And, in tears yet again in the pool before breakfast, and so castigating myself, I have to remind myself that she's only been dead for seven months and three days.

And William Fiennes' brother also died. He had a fit aged 41 from which he didn't recover. He stopped breathing instead. One of the most enduring memories is of Richard reciting a long poem from memory to an audience in the music room, all holding their breath willing him to finish it, and finish it well. He did. He was happy; he glowed in their applause. Sadly, by the time of his death, the violence and outbursts had long disappeared; he was content in his new centre, valued by the staff, and working as a gardener. He had his own important routines, such as smoking a pipe, and moreover, Leeds United were on the up. I guess he left when the party was in full swing. His parents had had another loss, a boy named Thomas who died aged only three.

'Richard was buried beside Thomas. "We are rich in what we have lost," my mother said, in the kitchen. She wasn't sure where the words had come from, but she kept repeating them, hearing his name in them: "We are rich in what we have lost. We are rich."'

And indeed, I know too that whatever comes next, I am rich in what I have lost.

Epilogue: Those Really Final Words

August 2014 and I was at the Pride march in Leeds a few days ago. I was telling some much younger friends that the first march I went on was for the Gay Liberation Front in the mid-1970s, in London. We felt brave, frightened and excited. The onlookers were incredulous, hostile, and so utterly different from the carnival atmosphere in Leeds. Now lots of major corporations have a presence in the parade – Asda, Tesco, the NHS. These young friends said, 'Wow! It's because of you we have all this now!' Things have changed so much.

The day after, I read in the *Guardian* of an Anglican priest, Jeremy Pemberton, who had his offer of a job as an NHS chaplain withdrawn the day after he married his long-term partner. The problem is with his Bishop and there needs to be a 'two year discussion process within the Church' to allow people to marry same-sex partners.

Two men have said they love each other; Church panics.

OK, we are the love that dares speak its name; we say loudly, proudly, that our love is just as valid and beautiful as that of anyone else. We will still say so even if we are beaten with sticks and beaten with words. We will stand up in public, get married, and we will say it at each other's funerals. This is what I said at yours:

Letter to Irene from Rach at her funeral:

Well, this is it – my goodbyes. Irene. My partner of 33 years.

I'm not quite sure what to say to you now, how to sum it up, except that I wouldn't have missed it for the world. What a ride you have given me.

Your descent into Alzheimer's broke my heart. I don't know if it will mend fully but I will try, for your sake, and I know you would want me to be happy. I have picked up my life but still, so often it feels strange without you. It's nearly six years since you had to leave home and I have visited you faithfully, sometimes reluctantly, sometimes joyfully, and always I have carried something away too, some speck of love that you still hold for me, and still managed to show, a testament to how love does indeed conquer all, showing through, somehow, from the heart that was still there despite the damaged brain.

We did such a lot together, you and I. So many of the memories are mine alone now, long gone from your mind. The epic walks we did are what most come into my mind, real shared feats of endurance and so many fantastic views, mountains, trees, sunsets, mornings waking up in a tent in the wilderness. They were tough and we did them together. A shared life – what more could I ask for? You were my soul mate, a true love. We had so much in common, and a lovely home, good friends, close family, and more love between us than many people have in a lifetime of partners, lovers…

I was so lucky to have met you. You were funny, intelligent, witty, sensitive. You taught me to love, and understand, Shakespeare, poetry, theatre, the Lake District, Scotland, and of course, our beloved Yorkshire. My goodness, we walked so much of it. You loved me, which fills me still with wonder, and I flourished because of your love. You showed it in your eyes when you saw me. And for me, I was always happy to see you at the end of a day; you were the centre of my world. We loved each other with all our hearts. How I loved you, my funny Valentine.

A little while ago I came back from a few nights away and as I walked through the arrival gates at Leeds Bradford Airport I saw so clearly, in my mind's eye, you standing there, waiting for me, a smile on your face. You weren't there, of course, and my eyes filled with tears. Sometimes, from nowhere, the memory of you ambushes me, and your presence comes into my present. I have learnt to live with your absence, with missing you – no longer every waking moment, but often; the loss of you fills my heart and I have worked hard not to let the sadness of your loss make me ache. What I would give to have you still here, well, whole and enjoying life.

You were always faster than me on your bike, and you would wait at the top of a hill for me to catch up. We loved cycling on our identical bikes and even a few weeks before you left home for the last time we were cycling in Holland. Amazing how we managed to do so much right to the end, even though your disease was so advanced. You have taken me to places I never thought I'd go – the care homes, hospitals. I never thought our lives and our partnership would end up in the way it did. It has all added to the richness and all in the end is harvest, but I would have loved to have grown old with you, to see how your older years and a happy retirement might have panned out. I wonder what sort of person you would have become if you hadn't been ill. I lost you in your fifties. We had such a hard decade as the dementia progressed and looking back I don't know how I managed. I did it for you, just as you would have done it for me.

In some ways your dying hasn't made such a difference as you are always with me, always were.

I don't know where you are now, but I know that you are waiting for me on the top of the hill.

Love you forever, Irene; sleep tight.

The story of Rachael and Irene inspired the play **'Don't Leave Me Now'** which explores the impact of early onset dementia on two very different families. Where does love end and duty begin – or does it? The play has been performed more than 60 times throughout the UK and Northern Ireland, always with a post-performance discussion. It is available to hospitals, hospices, universities, community groups, libraries and Local Authorities as well as to theatres for performances. The professional cast of five recreate parts of Irene and Rachael's story, interwoven with the story of Cindy and Chris who were also on the dementia journey together.

For further information please visit www.dontleavemenow.co.uk or on Facebook Don't Leave Me Now'. Contact Brian Daniels directly brdan@icloud.com.

Further Reading

Barnes, Julian. *Levels of Life.* London: Jonathan Cape, 2013.
Armstrong, Lance. *It's Not About the Bike.* New York: G.P. Putnam's Sons, 2000.
Bayley, John. *Iris: A Memoir of Iris Murdoch.* London: Gerald Duckworth & Co, 1998.
Didion, Joan. *The Year of Magical Thinking.* New York: Alfred A. Knopf, 2005.
Diamond, John. *C: Because Cowards Get Cancer Too.* London: Vermillion, 1998.
Ironsides, Virginia. *You'll Get Over It: The Rage of Bereavement.* London: Hamish Hamilton, 1996.
In Loving Memory. A Collection for Memorial Services, Funerals and Just Getting By, ed. Sally Emerson. London: Little, Brown, 2004.
Kraeplin, Emil. *Psychiatrie.* Leipzig: Ambr. Abel, 1887.
Leader, Darian. *The New Black: Mourning, Melancholia and Depression.* London: Hamish Hamilton, 2008.
Lewis, C.S. *A Grief Observed.* London: Faber & Faber, 2013.
Oates, Joyce Carol. *The Falls.* New York: HarperCollins, 2004.
Walker, Alice. *Now Is the Time to Open Your Heart.* New York: Random House, 2004.

Useful Contacts

Alzheimer's Society
www.alzheimers.org.uk

Alzheimer's Support
www.alzheimerswiltshire.org.uk

Admiral Nurses
www.dementiauk.org

Stonewall
www.stonewall.org.uk

Alzheimer's Research UK
www.alzheimersresearchuk.org

LGBT Foundation
lgbt.foundation

BRACE: Funding Research Into Alzheimer's
www.alzheimers-brace.org

London Friend: LGBT health and wellbeing
www.londonfriend.org.uk

Alzheimer Scotland: Action on Dementia
www.alzcot.org

Age UK
www.ageuk.org.uk

nauteus

nausea